W9-BZP-797

THE LITTLE RED BOOK OF
RUNNING

THE LITTLE RED BOOK OF
RUNNING

SCOTT DOUGLAS

FOREWORD BY AMBY BURFOOT

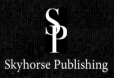

Skyhorse Publishing

Skyhorse Publishing books may be purchased in bulk at special discounts for sales promotion, corporate gifts, fund-raising, or educational purposes. Special editions can also be created to specifications. For details, contact the Special Sales Department, Skyhorse Publishing, 307 West 36th Street, 11th Floor, New York, NY 10018 or info@skyhorsepublishing.com.

Skyhorse® and Skyhorse Publishing® are registered trademarks of Skyhorse Publishing, Inc.®, a Delaware corporation.

www.skyhorsepublishing.com

10 9 8 7 6 5 4 3 2 1

Library of Congress Cataloging-in-Publication Data is available on file.
ISBN: 978-1-61608-296-3

Printed in China

To the hundreds of fellow runners who have shared the road and their thoughts with me over the last three decades. Thanks for the run!

Contents

PART TWO
Running Faster: 63 Tips to Help Build Your Speed, Even If You're Never Going to Race

PART THREE
Running Injury-Free: 50 Tips to Help You Avoid, Treat, and Beat Injuries

PART FOUR
Running Consistently: 43 Tips to Help You Run More Often for the Rest of Your Life

PART FIVE
Running Miscellany: 49 Tips on Shoes and Safety, Attitude and Altitude, and Everything Else That Matters

Acknowledgments

Thanks to Bill Wolfsthal of Skyhorse Publishing for bringing this project to life; to Amby Burfoot for honoring me by writing the foreword; to Meredith Freimer for listening to me babble on about this book during long runs together; and to the photographers whose work herein captures the spirit of enjoyable running: Jonathan Beverly, Stacey Cramp, Brian Metzler, Alison Wade, and Joel Wolpert.

Foreword

When I was a kid, one of my favorite books was *The Little Engine That Could.* As a high school runner and beyond, I often recalled the "I think I can, I think I can" message of the book, especially on seemingly long hills. It sounds so silly, but the message was motivating for me long before I knew other expressions of a similar theme. It was a simple little thing that helped me more than a hundred-page treatise on sports psychology ever could.

In high school, I had the good fortune to be coached by John J. Kelley, a two-time Olympian and the winner of the 1957 Boston Marathon. In many hours at his kitchen table, I heard endless quotes from his fellow New England skeptic, Henry David Thoreau. One was "Our life is frittered away by detail. Simplify, simplify." This one had a strong effect. I took it to mean that I didn't have to do a lot of talking or thinking to be a good runner. I just had to do the work.

Running is simple. When we keep it that way, we generally have the best chance of enjoying it and reaching our goals. Often, it's a little nugget of wisdom, or a way to think about something, that's more helpful than a day-by-day six-month training program handed down from Mount Olympus. That's certainly been my experience, from high school to winning the 1968 Boston Marathon and in the decades since as I've made the inevitable adjustments to age. A few words from a trusted source who's been in your shoes go a long way.

That's what you have here with *The Little Red Book of Running*. Scott Douglas has an encyclopedic knowledge of running, and the clarity of mind to simplify, simplify and pass on the essential information. I'm sure you'll find many of the tips in this book to be just what you need to get the most out of your running at different points in your running life.

Amby Burfoot
Editor at Large, *Runner's World*
1968 Boston Marathon Champion

Introduction

I wrote this book during the winter of 2010/2011, but I've been working on it since 1979.

That's the year when, as a ninth grader, I started running. Immediately I was enamored. I loved the sense of exploration, of challenging myself, of being outside in all kinds of weather. I loved the time alone, time to think about whatever came to my head. I loved seeing if I could go farther than I ever had, or run a loop faster than I did the week before. I loved how I felt physically while running and how I felt mentally when I was done.

When I joined the high school cross-country team that fall, I learned to love running even more. Training with friends, racing against those friends, building toward a long-term goal—all this and more about being a competitive runner added a whole other layer of attraction to this most natural act.

In that first year of running, I sought to learn as much about the sport as I could. I went to the library and checked out every book and magazine I could find. (Little did I know I would one day work for one of them.) I pestered my coach nonstop about workouts and mileage and racing strategies. I asked my team-mates about what running felt like to them to see what I could take from their experiences and apply it to my situation. When I started road racing later that year, I talked with anyone who would spare a few minutes: How much did they run? How fast? What was their favorite workout? What did they do when their knee hurt, or it was hot, or snowing? What did they eat the night before a race? And a million other questions about the little things that can have such a big effect on running.

Throughout high school, college, and then when running on my own after school, I kept talking to pretty much any runner I thought I could learn from. Eventually, starting in the early 1990s, I found my way into writing about running. Now I suddenly was talking with some of the best runners and coaches in the world, and I took full advantage of the opportunity. Through applying what I learned and a dedicated but not obsessive work ethic, I was able to run above-average times, such as 30:48 for 10K and 51:01 for 10 miles, that were much faster than I "should" have run given my fairly average natural talent.

I've been fortunate enough to learn from hundreds of world-class distance runners and coaches through talking with them, observing them, and running with them. By now it's become second nature to take what I learn from those encounters and run it through the filter I first used in high school: How can I use this information to make my running more enjoyable and successful? And by extension, via magazine articles and the four books on running I've coauthored, how can I share this information with my fellow runners at all levels so that they, too, can get more out of their running?

The result of the last three decades of this curiosity is this book. It's not meant to be the ultimate treatise on running or a day-by-day guide to peak performance. If I've learned anything over the last three decades, it's that success in running often comes from one or two tweaks to your training or mind-set. This book is full of little such nuggets that can have large positive effects. I hope you find its distilled wisdom useful in making your running more enjoyable, satisfying, and a regular highlight of your life.

Scott Douglas
Senior Editor, *Running Times*

PART ONE

Running More:
45 Tips to Help You Safely and Successfully Increase Your Daily and Weekly Mileage

"How much do you run?"

Every runner has been asked that question, even from non-runners. It's an implicit acknowledgment that when we think about running, we fundamentally think in terms of volume, both for individual runs and for longer blocks of time. "How much do you run?" can mean on an average day, or how many times a week, or how many miles per week, or how many hours a week. You could even answer the question (and blow the questioner's mind) by saying something like, "Last year, I ran 2,715 miles. That was down a few hundred from the year before because I had a calf strain in February and some hamstring issues in the fall."

So the first thing most runners want to know is how to handle running more. After all, even if your main goal in running is to see how fast you can run, first you need to be able to cover the distance. And you need to be able to cover that distance reasonably comfortably so that you're good to go on the next run, and the one after that, building that baseline of fitness you need for running to be enjoyable.

At some point, every runner gets to what seems to be their running set point, in one or more of the ways to answer "How much do you run?" It might be the length of the average run, or the duration of the longest run, or number of runs per week, or miles run per week or month or year. It's fine to stay at that set point, of course, but most runners want more. (You wouldn't have become a runner in the first place if you're the sort who's easily contented.) The tips in this chapter are about how to get past those set points. They're about how to advance your fitness by running more, whether that's on a daily, weekly, or yearly basis.

1

A Crucial Opening Thought

There are no junk miles. You may have heard otherwise from well-meaning people. Junk miles, they'll tell you, are miles that you do just to do, maybe to reach a more impressive weekly mileage figure, maybe just because you've noticed that good runners tend to run a lot and you've therefore concluded that more is better. Junk miles, they'll say, are wasted time, because they don't help you reach your running goals.

Don't believe them. Allow me to repeat: There are no junk miles. If you're not injured so badly that you're altering your form, or so sick that you feel much worse after running, then it's all good.

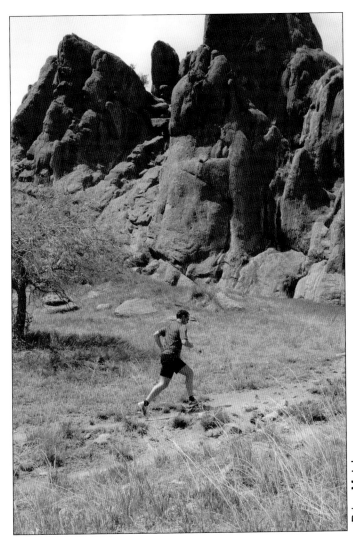

: Brian Metzler

People who warn of junk miles often point out the law of diminishing returns. "After x number of miles per week," they'll say, "the benefit from any one run really starts to decline." And they're right. But diminishing returns are still returns. If you're motivated enough to run a little extra in search of a little more fitness, have at it.

Even if you think a run doesn't advance your fitness, it has other benefits—promoting blood flow, clearing your mind, getting you away from the computer, burning calories, getting you out in nature, helping you spend time with friends, giving you much-needed time by yourself, maintaining the rhythm of good training, and infinitely so on. These aspects of running that have little to do with peak performance are usually ignored by people warning of junk miles. There a million reasons to go for a run today that have nothing to do with running faster next weekend. The more of them that appeal to you, the less reason there is to believe in junk miles.

2

A Crucial Second Thought

Let me be clear from the outset: I'm not saying that more running is always better, either for your running performance or the rest of your life. Obviously there's a point where running more is an overall negative.

But most of us are never at risk of reaching that point. Even among longtime ambitious runners, most of us are in shape to get in shape—we've never really tested the limits of our running potential. And that's fine. Certainly most of us have several other claims on our time and energy, and working twice as hard to improve another 10 percent as a runner might not make sense to you.

But it doesn't follow from that acknowledgment that anything more than what you've become used to is a waste of time, or that experimenting with bumping up your set point will inevitably lead to injury or burnout. How do you know if you've never tried? Again, no one is saying you have to try. But if you want to, don't be scared off by vague warnings of "overtraining" or "staleness." Yes, when you try to push past your current limits, you might get tired. That will pass. As long as you go about advancing your running fitness intelligently, you can avoid injury while becoming fitter than you might have thought possible.

3

The First Step in Running More

Slow down. Most people who feel stuck at a certain level of running are simply running too many of their runs too fast.

Try this thought experiment: Let's say you want to tack on an additional 15 minutes to most of your daily runs. Would you be able to do so by doing your normal run and then sprinting for 15 minutes? No. Would you be able to do so by doing your normal run and then walking for 15 minutes? Of course. Would you be able to do so by doing your normal run and then continuing on at that pace for 15 minutes? Probably, but it would be difficult, and if you tried to do it every time you ran, you'd either start to be unable to hold the pace or you wouldn't even try because every run would have become too much of a challenge. So the right pace

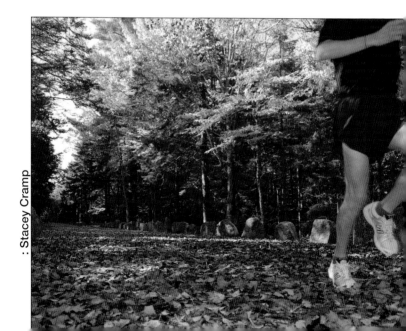

: Stacey Cramp

in this scenario is somewhere between a walk and a little slower than your current normal pace.

Apply that thinking to your running as a whole when you want to run more. If you want to run more on each run, run at least the first half of the run slower than you do now. If you want to run more days per week, run each day a little slower than you have been when running fewer days per week.

4

The Right Effort for Running More

In saying to slow down to best be able to handle more running, I'm not talking about minutes per mile slower than normal. I mean to ease back from your usual effort level to where you have a good balance between feeling like you're running with your normal form and feeling like your perceived effort is lower than usual. You should have the feeling of storing up energy more than slowly leaking it. As opposed to the feeling of "I could keep going at this pace if I had to, but I'd rather not, and anything much faster would be a real strain," aim for "I could keep going at this pace for at least as long as I've been out, and if I had to pick it up for the next 5 minutes, I could easily handle that."

When you're trying to bump up your mileage, be mindful of your breathing. It should be easy and light throughout these runs. Let the duration be the limiting factor. That will be manifested more in muscular fatigue, the sign that you're properly pushing your limits ever so slightly. If you're breathing hard for most of the run, you're never going to be able to run far enough to reach that desired state of muscular fatigue.

First cover the distance. Then worry about covering it faster.

5

When Trying to Run More, Let the Pace Come to You

The best way to be at the proper gentle effort when you're trying to run more is to start more slowly than you think is necessary. Instead of forcing things so that you're at the pace you "should" be by the time you've gone around the block, start at a trot. As your heart rate increases gradually and your muscles start to warm up from a gently increasing blood flow, you'll naturally feel like running faster, without even having to think, "OK, now I feel ready to run faster." Within 10 or 15 minutes, you'll find that you're running much faster with almost no increase in your perceived effort.

6

In Fact, Always Let the Pace Come to You

Even if you're not trying to run more, start out a lot slower than you'll be running when you finish. Easing into runs and gradually picking up the pace as feels comfortable is one of the keys to making more runs enjoyable and fruitful.

This isn't how most of us go about it, of course. We have an idea how fast we "should" be running, and we do our damndest to get to that pace as quickly as possible. Otherwise, we think, we're wasting our time. We think we're almost cheating, like we're not working hard enough to get in a real workout.

7

Take a Lesson from Kenyans

A few years ago I spent a month in one of Kenya's running hotbeds. Every run I did there with Kenyans began at a glorified stumble. On the first few, I couldn't believe how slowly we were going. And this was with some of the best runners in the world—two of the guys I did several runs with have broken 13:00 for 5K, and many of the high school students I ran with have represented Kenya in international competitions.

Inevitably, the pace quickened. But it did so organically, not because someone checked her watch a mile into the run and said, "We're running too slow, we better pick it up." Over the first 15 or so minutes, I could tell we were running faster, but my effort level was the same. (We were running at 8,000 feet of elevation, and I live by the ocean in Maine, so I was acutely aware throughout my trip of the effects of altitude on my perceived effort.) By the last third of the run, we would be out and out moving, with the last few minutes at close to a race level of effort.

I'm certainly not saying to finish every run at a sprint. But these runs in Kenya were a revelation: There was never a point in the run where you could say, "Ah, now it's suddenly gotten harder." Day after day, some of the best runners in the world let their bodies tell them when it was time to go slow and when it was time to indulge in faster running.

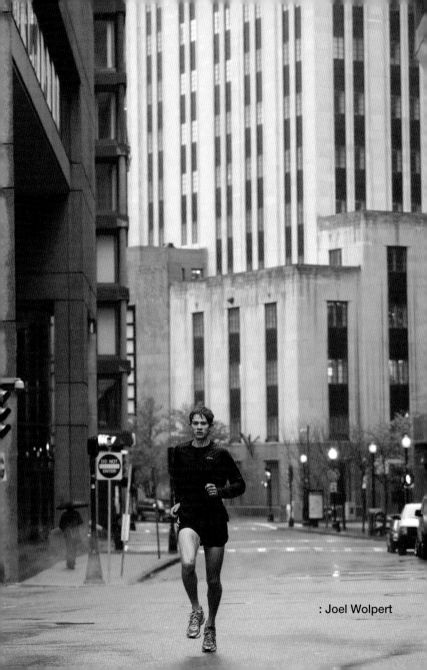

: Joel Wolpert

8
Strength Builds Speed

Another thing to keep in mind if you think you're running too slowly for it to be worthwhile: Your basic aerobic fitness is the main determinant of how fast or slow feels comfortable on a typical daily run. The fitter you are, the faster will feel comfortable. And for almost everyone reading this book, the best way to advance that fitness is to run more, rather than your normal amount at a faster pace. As you get fitter through more mileage, what feels like a comfortable everyday pace will eventually become faster. By slowing a bit now while building your mileage, later you'll be running more, and at a faster pace, than might seem conceivable now.

9
The No-Brainer Approach to Running More

Out-and-back courses are a great way to sort of trick yourself into extending individual runs. If your goal for the day is to run for an hour, head out for 30 minutes before you turn around for home. You're pretty much guaranteed to succeed. You'll probably still feel fresh at the turnaround, and then there are no temptations to overcome in the second half when you're more tired, as can be the case if you're doing a loop that has ways to shorten it or you add on by running past your house with 12 minutes to go.

10

More Days of Running or More Running Per Day?

When you're trying to up your mileage, should you run more often or run more on the days you run?

The best answer to that specific question is a general answer that applies to so much of running: Do whatever is more likely to more often lead to success.

11

Now for More Specifics

If you're running a few days a week, is that for time reasons? If so—for example, if there are only three days a week where you currently can find the time to run, but have a bit of wiggle room in those windows of opportunity—then run more on your running days. If your schedule is super crammed, you'll probably more regularly run more by adding 15 minutes to each run than by carving out a devoted-to-running block of time on another day.

If you're running a few days a week but could find the time on other days, then start by adding another day of running each week, and keep the distance of your normal runs the same. Once you adapt to the increased workload (which probably won't take more than a few weeks), weeks with four days of running, or five days, or whatever the new amount is, will feel like the new normal.

If you already run pretty much every day, then start adding additional mileage to your medium-effort days of the week. On days when you do hard workouts, you could add a mile or two to each of your warm-up and cool-down. Then you could make your longest run of the week a little longer. Tack on mileage on these days before running more on your easiest days; keep those really easy so that they serve as true recovery days instead of becoming another medium-effort day.

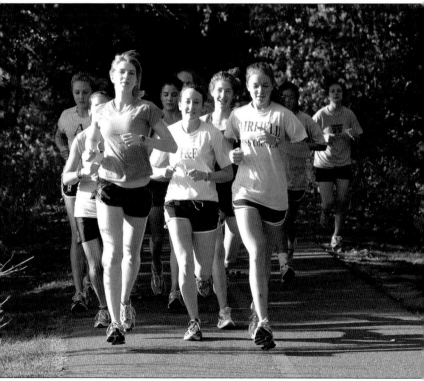

: Alison Wade

12

Keeping Track

Every runner even slightly interested in performance should keep a running log. Unless you have an amazing memory, you'll benefit from recording what you ran when before it slips out of mind. Over time your log will reveal patterns that can guide future decisions, such as how many days it takes you to feel recovered from a hard workout or which types of workouts seem to consistently lead to a given body ache. Logs are also great for reminding yourself how you trained before a given performance so that you can have objective information on what you needed to do to reach that level and insights on how to exceed it.

Include in your log whatever details from runs are necessary for you to be able to benefit from entries upon review. In addition to distance and/or time, that could include the type of course, the weather, time of day, what else happened in your life that day, etc. Beyond the basics, I always note anything that made the run different: Did it have a lot of downhills? Then that's worth putting in so that if two days later my quads are really sore I have an obvious explanation. Did I do a track workout? Then my times from it will help me know what to shoot for in future workouts. Was it really hot for my long run, and did I then plug away as per usual on subsequent days? Then a couple weeks later I might have an explanation if I've been feeling flat. Was work crazy the last week? Did I sleep poorly? Did I run with Jim and go faster than usual? Anything from the run that might affect you on subsequent runs is worth recording.

13
Log On Regularly

For your log to serve its purpose as a training tool, you should write in it at least a few times a week. Sitting down and rehashing your running twice a month isn't going to lead to a log that helps you discern patterns and learn from mistakes.

It's also helpful to keep track of longer-term matters, such as weekly mileage and a monthly summary of miles, number of days run, number of stretching sessions, things like that. Having these details recorded keeps you honest—it can be easy to think you've done more than you have.

Good information on your long-term patterns is also helpful because success in running comes not from occasional great days, but by steady progress over time. The principles that underlie successful long-term financial investment apply to running.

14
Minutes or Miles?

Whether you keep track of your running by miles run or time run doesn't matter as long as you have a system you use consistently that works for you.

Most people keep track by counting miles. That's true even for people who keep track of individual runs by minutes (e.g., "I ran for 42 minutes today, so it's going in the log as 5 miles"). Even though it has no intrinsic meaning to the human body, a mile is our standard unit of measurement, so we might as well go with it. (An American friend who lived in Europe for a couple of years started tracking his running in kilometers and jokingly noted how much more fun it was to say, "I've been hitting 150 a week" than, "I've been doing 90 a week.")

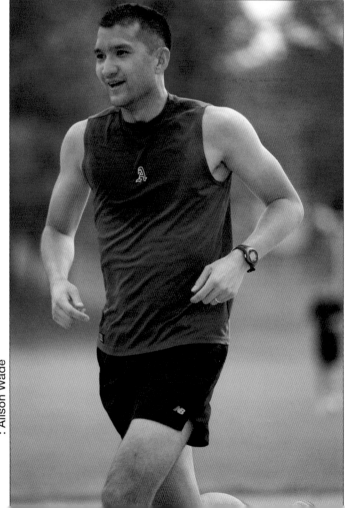

: Alison Wade

15

Rough Estimates

Most of your runs are going to be guesstimations based on how fast you think you typically run and how long it takes you to cover one of your courses on average. When improvising a course, you're relying totally on what general pace you think you're running that day. And that's fine—it really doesn't matter if what you say is your 10-mile loop is 9.8 miles long, or if you call a run 5 miles when it's longer than that.

Online mapping tools can be useful to see how far your courses are. Don't get too hung up on their degree of accuracy—I've seen the same program give a different distance for the same course on consecutive days. They also aren't going to measure a course exactly as you ran it, and they don't account for things like hills and wind. So be content with getting a close-enough measurement.

When in doubt, err on the side of underestimating. It's more common to think we're running farther and faster than we really are than it is to shortchange ourselves.

16

Keep Gadgets in Their Place

The top runners who lean heavily on gadgets like a GPS system are the exceptions. Most elites have their courses, assign a distance to each, and leave it at that. They're secure enough in their running that they don't need the constant external feedback from a Garmin or similar gadget. They know that what matters on a run is achieving a certain effort for a certain duration. Most of the time they base that on the signals they're getting from their bodies, not from a potentially faulty device on their wrist.

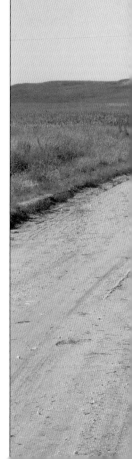

Granted, it can be nice occasionally to know exactly how far you ran at what pace. GPS units are great if you're doing something like a long run with the last several miles at your goal marathon race pace. That's valuable feedback about your progress toward a specific goal that combines the elements of time and distance.

But too many runners overrely on their measuring gadgets during normal runs, when it's not important to hit specific combinations of time and distance. To them, a run is successful only if the gadget spits out the right numbers. It's worth making this point again: A mile has no meaning to the human body. You're imposing artificial definitions of success on your running by letting a device that speaks only in those measurements tell you if you had a good run. Learn to distinguish between information about your running that has merit and information about your running that's just information for the sake of information. Learn to interpret and be guided by the signals from your body about proper effort levels.

: 101° West

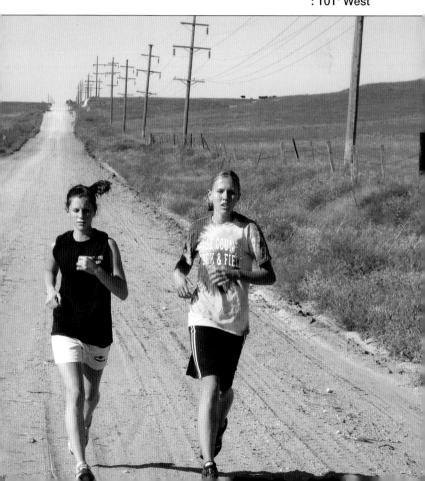

17

Be an Honest Accountant

Whatever your system, keep it on the up and up. Padding your log to produce more impressive figures serves no purpose other than self-delusion. You can tell yourself you've been running x number of miles per week all you want, but if you're consistently getting to x via fuzzy math, what's the point? Your body will tell you it's really been less than x, especially when it comes time to race. (Besides, if you can't be honest with yourself about how much you've been running, in what other ways are you deceiving yourself?)

One Olympic marathoner I know specialized in inflating his log. He'd be out with a group on, say, a 10-miler, and say, "Hey, guys, let's slow it down, I want to get 11 for the day." That is, he was going to run the same distance, but by making the run take more time, he then allowed himself to count the run as farther. He even claimed in a running magazine that putting down that he'd run 120 miles for a week instead of the 100 he probably ran gave him more confidence. I've yet to find anyone else in the fifteen years since he stated this who thought it was a good idea.

18

Some Days, Leave the Watch at Home

At least a few days a week, decide what course you're going to run, and then leave your watch at home. Other days, run wherever, guided by total time on your watch. The thing to mostly avoid is timing yourself over the same courses day after day. That way lies the madness of beating yourself up for running slower than you "should" or forcing yourself to pick it up because you're 6 seconds slower at your 45-minutes-into-it checkpoint than you were yesterday.

19

Increasing Weekly Mileage

At some point, "running more" pretty much becomes "increasing weekly mileage," because that's how most runners track things.

Weekly mileage might not be the best framing device for tracking how much you run. You might make the common mistake of viewing each week as its own entity, with things that "have" to happen in that week for the week to be successful. Similarly, you might tend to view your training primarily in blocks of a week, rather than a broader view that more accurately reflects how your body responds to the stimulus of running. Tracking monthly mileage so that you don't artificially force certain things to happen within each horizontal strip of a calendar might be a more prudent approach.

But most of the rest of our lives are shaped by the week's seven-day cycle, so it makes some sense for a week to be the next unit of training after a day.

20

Ignore the 10 Percent "Rule"

You've probably heard that, when upping your running volume, you shouldn't increase your mileage by more than 10 percent a week. You have not only my permission but my encouragement to ignore this "rule."

For starters, as I've mentioned, the unit of a mile has no meaning to the human body. Neither does the seven-day cycle we call a week. Neither does the base-10 number system, our use of which is where the "rule" comes from. (Did the Babylonian coaches of antiquity dole out advice about increasing volume in units of 60 because they happened to grow up using a base-60

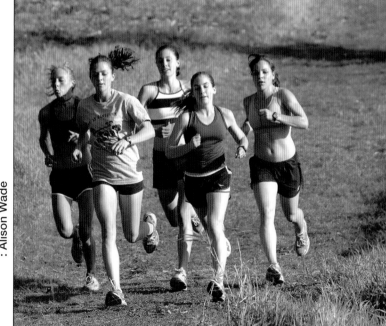

number system?) So it stands to reason that combining these three variables doesn't make for any sort of sound guidance.

Even if the intent of the "rule" is more right than wrong—i.e., increase your running volume gradually to allow your body to adapt—its literal application can have comical consequences. Say someone is running 4 miles a day, 3 days a week. He decides he wants to run more than 12 miles per week. He's in good health, has no injury problems, and simply wants to run more to feel that much better and get fitter. Applying the 10 percent formula, he would move to 13.2 miles per week, then 14.5, then 15.9, and finally 17.4 by the end of the month. For most people, this is like locking your house every time you go next door to borrow an egg—safe, certainly, but verging into letting fear of something bad happening overwhelm everything else.

21

A Better Way to Increase Weekly Mileage

If most weeks you're running less than four times, then simply add another day of running, with the distance toward the shorter end of what you usually run. So in our example above, our hero could add a fourth day of running to his week and immediately be at 16 miles per week. As I noted earlier, keep the pace easy on both the new run and existing ones.

If you run most days of the week and aren't interested in additional runs, then add a mile or two, or 10 to 20 minutes, to each run in a week.

22

Hold On to Your New Mileage Level

And now here's the important thing: Hold that new level for two or three weeks. Give your body time to adapt to the new stress. This is another area where the 10 percent formula falls short. As infinitesimal as some of the increases it can lead to are, they're still increases. Your body never has a chance to adapt to the new workload before you throw another increase at it.

Let's say you're running 30 miles a week. Instead of going from 30 miles a week to 33.3 to 36.6 to 40.2, jump up immediately to 40, then hold at 40 a week for two or three weeks.

23

Down Weeks

Here's the second key to increasing weekly mileage in a safe but meaningful way: Take occasional down weeks before lighting out for the next milestone.

In the example from above, you've gone from 30 to 40 miles a week all at once, then held that new level for two or three weeks. Now, go back down to the weekly mileage you used to run; in this case, follow a few 40-mile weeks with a 30-mile week. This "down week" will give your body a chance to consolidate the gains you made in increasing your mileage. During the down week, keep most runs easy, even if you start to feel raring to go by the end of the week. Save that energy for when you return to your new higher level of mileage.

After the down week, you could either hold at your new level for a few more weeks, or take another leap in mileage, like up to 45 a week for a couple of weeks before taking a down week of 35–40 miles. Keep working this stress-and-recovery approach to your weeks as a whole until you're at the level of mileage your body, mind, and outside life agree is best.

24

When More Is Too Much

Expect to feel tired when you first move up to a new level of mileage. The sensation you'll likely have will be of your legs feeling a little heavier or deader. It might take you a bit longer on runs to feel like you're in a good rhythm. You might feel a little lethargic during your non-running hours. Increased (or oddly, decreased) appetite might also accompany a bump up in mileage.

These signs are normal and will pass if you haven't increased your mileage too quickly. Some signs that you've taken on more than you can currently handle: New acute running-related pains (as opposed to some generalized soreness or tightness); a precipitous drop in your performance (as opposed to being a little slower, which you should purposefully do anyway); and/or otherwise inexplicable signs of a cold or other illness. If any of these accompany your increased mileage, go back down to your previous mileage until they pass. Then shoot for a new higher mileage level that's below your first attempt at an increase.

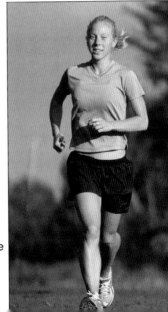

: Alison Wade

25

25

Add New Stresses Judiciously

If at all possible, time attempts at increasing your mileage for when the rest of your life is on a relatively even keel. Your chances of adapting to the new running stress will be greater if the increased mileage doesn't coincide with your crazy time at work or a family crisis or absolutely atrocious weather.

26

Love the Long Run

Doing one run a week that's significantly longer than most of your other runs is a great way to simultaneously boost your mileage and your fitness. Your main motivation for regularly doing long runs should be the latter—building your endurance so that all of your runs become more manageable. But I'm not going to deny that starting the week with a long run is a killer kick-off to meeting your weekly mileage goal.

Near-weekly long runs are, of course, one of the backbones of marathon-training plans. Almost all runners looking to race well from 5K on up know the value of the long run. The internal changes in your muscles caused by long runs—basically, a vastly improved "plumbing" system for getting oxygen to and removing waste products from working muscles—carry over to all your runs. There's also a great mental benefit from these runs devoted to making yourself more resistant to fatigue, in that your normal runs won't seem nearly as daunting. When you're used to a 2-hour run most weeks, a 45-minute run on even the most stressful day of the week is easy to imagine.

27

How Long Is Long?

For people who run almost daily, a long run should be between 20 percent and 30 percent of your total weekly mileage. So if you run 40 miles per week, have one run a week be at least 8 and up to 12 miles long.

Another general guideline is for your long run to be at least one-third longer than any other run that week. This guideline is more useful for people who run a moderate amount a few days a week. So if you typically run 5 miles four days a week, lengthen one of those to closer to 7 miles. It's fine to cut back one of the other runs if you want to stay at the same weekly mileage. You'll gain more fitness by varying the lengths of your runs.

28

How Long Is Too Long?

If your longest run of the week is more than twice the distance of any other run in a typical week, it's too long. This is one of the problems with the training programs used by many first-time marathoners—they quickly bump up their long run, and soon it constitutes the bulk of their weekly mileage. The run is so long relative to what their bodies are used to that they spend the rest of the week recovering from it and do just a couple token jogs. In this case, the solution is to bring the runs in a week more in line with each other. Bump up your weekly mileage by making one of the other runs during the week longer, and get your longest run of the week back down to no more than twice as long as any other run you do.

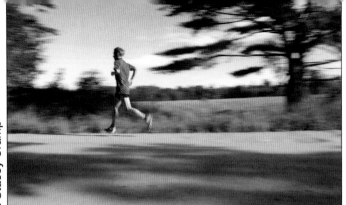

: Stacey Cramp

29

Making Long Runs Longer

To bump up your long runs, try adding 1 or 2 miles per long run for two consecutive long runs, then come down every third long run to your earlier distance. So if your long run is currently 12 miles and you want to increase it, you could go to 13 for the next one, then 14 the one after that, but then back down to 12 for the next one. This will better allow you to adapt to the longer long runs than plowing ahead with longer and longer ones week after week.

30

When to Go Long

Whenever! The weekend long run is a staple in most training programs, but nowhere is it written in stone that you can't go long on Tuesday morning or Thursday evening. For most people on a normal work schedule, a weekend morning is the easiest place to find the time. But have I impressed upon you yet the great value in not tying your running to artificial parameters? Good, then feel free to go long whenever works for you.

Along those lines, there's nothing saying you have to go long every 7 days. Perhaps you'll find a 5-day training cycle works better for you. Or maybe you'll find that weekends are indeed the only time you have to go long, but doing so every weekend is simply too much, either for your body or your outside life. That's fine. If you can get in two or three long runs most months, you're getting enough of the long-run stimulus to significantly boost your endurance.

31

Where to Go Long

If you can swing it logistically, do your long runs on your nicer routes. It's one thing to suck it up and run wherever when you're getting in a short run after a stressful workday. Try to make your long runs a more pleasant experience. With the extra distance, you get to roam farther afield than usual. Explore the places you don't get to as often.

Don't feel guilty about driving somewhere special for your long runs. Long runs in an aesthetically pleasing environment, like a network of trails, go by a lot more quickly mentally. Also, the more forgiving surface of a trail or dirt road will lessen the pounding on your legs and lengthen your time to fatigue.

Try to include some hills in your long runs. The extra work getting up them will result in more of the improvements to your plumbing system that you want from a long run. In addition, the slight change in form you'll use going up and down will spread the stress across more of your leg muscles and lengthen your time to fatigue. A long run on a pancake-flat course will have you running with the same form throughout and you'll probably tighten up sooner than on a route with more variety.

32

Make Your Long-Run Days Special

A nice course goes a long way (ha-ha) toward making a long run enjoyable. If you can, include other elements so that long-run days are ones you really look forward to. Run them with friends. Go out for brunch afterward. Schedule a massage. Have a soak in a hot tub or bath. Do them on unharried days so that you can relax afterward and enjoy that pleasantly fatigued mellow feeling.

Most days you're going to scramble to fit your running around the rest of your life. Try to have long runs be one of the center-pieces of your day once in a while. You'll be reminded of the many things you love about running.

33

How Fast on Long Runs?

If there were ever a type of run to ease into, it's the long run. When people have to slow at the end of a long run, or cut it short, it's almost always because they've run the first half of it too hard.

Fifteen minutes into a long run, you should be running no faster than the pace you can honestly tell yourself you can hold to the end. If you get to a few miles to go and are itching to pick up the pace, that's the time to run faster. There are few running experiences more unpleasant than crashing and crawling in the last third of a long run.

Unless your long run is a key part of preparation for a long race—which we'll look at in the next chapter—keep your pace at a relaxed, conversational effort throughout. The challenge is simply covering the distance. The range of effort at which the physiological changes you're after by going long is broad; increase your chances of finishing the long run feeling strong by keeping things at the gentler end of that broad range.

If you plan your training in terms of minutes per mile relative to race pace, try these rough guidelines: Do your long run a minute per mile or slower than your marathon race pace, or 90 seconds to 2 minutes per mile slower than your 5K race pace.

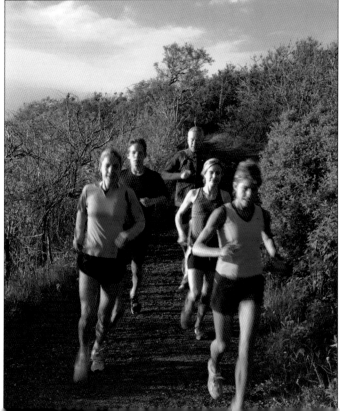

: Stacey Cramp

34

When a Long Run Isn't Going Well

Sometimes it's just not your day. When is it OK to pull the plug on a long run?

If you have an acute running-related pain that's getting worse as you run, stop. If you started the run with slight symptoms of a cold or illness and they're getting worse as you run, stop. (Easier said than done, of course, if these things happen when you're 5 miles from home. It's not against the law to ask to use someone's phone and call home for emergency taxi service.)

Other cases are more of a judgment call. If by "not going well" you mean you just don't feel like it, but you're fine physically, you should probably see it through. One of the benefits of long runs is learning to persevere mentally. Cutting a long run short because of a mental lapse will make it easier to make the same decision the next time it happens.

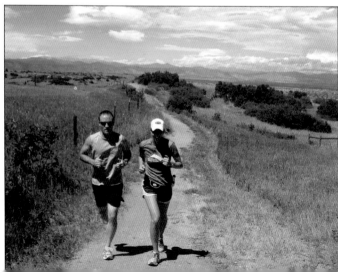

: Brian Metzler

Get through tough mental patches by breaking the run into smaller segments. Instead of obsessing over the fact that you still have an hour to go, concentrate on the next 10 minutes, then the 10 minutes after that. If you're running with a friend, get her talking. Ask about something you know will set her off; by the end of the anecdote, you'll be that much closer to home.

If your form is starting to deteriorate, it's OK to stop and collect yourself. Gently stretch areas that are tightening. Then ease back into the run. Sometimes the solution is to run a little faster, because that can get you running with better form. Try picking up the pace for a minute, then back off for a few minutes, then pick it up again for a minute.

If you started the run really tired and things haven't improved in the first hour, stick it out in most cases, but be aware that you're probably going to need some solid recovery time later that day. If things are such in the rest of your life that you need to be "on" for much of the rest of the day, then this might be a good day to cut your losses and try for long-run success another day.

If you've bonked and have to slow significantly the last few miles, finish it up, and resolve to start the next run better-fueled and at a more manageable pace.

35

It's a Run, Not a Feast

Most people don't need to take in calories on long runs.

One of the purposes of long runs is to slightly deplete your muscles' stores of glycogen, the stored form of carbohydrate that's their preferred fuel source for distance running. When you go long and run down your glycogen stores, your body adapts by becoming better at storing glycogen. This adaptation results in having a bigger gas tank for the next time you go long. Running low on glycogen also makes you more efficient at burning glycogen—at a given pace, you'll burn less glycogen and more fat. This adaptation means you can make your bigger gas tank last longer. These adaptations make you a better runner not only on long runs, but on all runs.

Those adaptations don't happen as readily when you take in calories every few miles, as many runners have started doing in recent years. Downing gel packets and energy bars throughout your long run will certainly help you not bonk. But by sparing your glycogen stores, they'll limit the long run's ability to make you a more efficient runner.

If you feel you can't get through your long run without repeatedly drinking sport drink and eating gels or bars, then you're trying to run too far for your current fitness. A well-trained runner should be able to get through 18 to 20 miles with no real decline in performance without having to take in lots of calories.

36

Pre–Long Run Nutrition

The real fueling for a long run takes place the day before, not during. Do yourself a favor and make sure you're starting your long run with a full gas tank. Eat a high-carbohydrate dinner. Because carbohydrate metabolism requires water to store what you ate, make sure you're well hydrated before you go to bed.

If you're going long first thing in the morning, experiment with what foods you can eat soon before running without stomach duress. You don't need much more than a few hundred calories, tops—this will help replenish the glycogen stores in your liver and brain that dipped while you slept. A little snack like a piece of dry toast and a banana will elevate your blood-sugar level so that you start the run feeling stronger.

Regardless of your taste for water in the morning, have a couple glasses. Your body will thank you over the last half hour of your long run.

37
The Whys of Post–Long Run Nutrition

After, not during, a long run is the time to take in frequent calories. In the first half hour after a long run, your muscles are extraordinarily receptive to refueling. Glycogen resynthesis occurs at three times the normal rate during this recovery window. After the first half hour, your muscles' receptivity to refueling starts to decline, but remains elevated for another 90 minutes.

This is important for two reasons. First, beginning to refuel while this above-and-beyond resynthesis is possible will induce your leg muscles to produce the desirable adaptations I described above. Given that causing these adaptations is one of the main reasons to go long, why wouldn't you want to reap the maximum benefit from your hard work?

Second, the sooner you start refueling, the faster you'll recover from your long run. It might not seem important at the time, but trust me, if you lag on

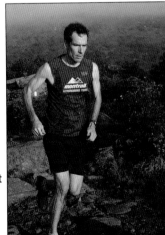

: Joel Wolpert

refueling after a Sunday long run, you might well be kicking your-self come Tuesday. When you're lackadaisical about post–long run nutrition, it's common to find yourself zapped later in the day. The next couple of days, you might realize you're more tired than you think you should be, and your enthusiasm for running will be low. You're also more likely to feel sore the day after a long run if you didn't start refueling soon enough.

38

The Whats of Post–Long Run Nutrition

The first order of business is rehydrating with water or sport drink. If your stomach tends to bother you after long runs, go with sport drink so that you're sure to get some calories in during that crucial first half hour after you finish.

Aim for a few hundred calories within 30 minutes of finishing. A carb-to-protein ratio of 4:1 at this time will increase glycogen resynthesis, so something like a bagel with hummus, peanut butter, tuna, or cheese works well if your stomach can tolerate it.

After the immediate aftermath, have a large carbohydrate-rich meal 2 two hours of finishing. Keep rehydrating throughout the day—if you find your energy lagging several hours after a long run and you refueled properly after, then it's probably because you're still dehydrated. If you have a headache later that day, that's also a sign of still being dehydrated.

Include a good source of protein with dinner to help with muscle tissue repair. Many people find a glass of red wine or a beer with dinner after a long run helps them sleep better, thereby furthering their recovery.

39
The Rest of Long-Run Recovery

There's more to optimizing recovery from a long run than eating. (Sorry.)

While you're rehydrating and refueling in the first half hour after, do some gentle stretches for any areas that got tight during the run. That's probably going to mean your hamstrings, hips, and lower back. This is especially important if you've driven to run and are about to get back in your car. If you drove, do more light stretching when you get home to undo sitting in the car while your muscles were compromised.

If you can find time later that day for a longer, more thorough stretching session, you'll speed your recovery. Ten to 15 minutes several hours later will increase blood flow and leave you feeling less beat up and laggardly the next day. A walk or swim that afternoon will serve the same purpose. You might not feel like these little extras are making much of a difference at the time, but they're guaranteed to contribute to your feeling better in the days after. That will allow you to maintain a better training rhythm and pile fitness gain upon fitness gain.

40
Double Your Endurance Pleasure

Here's a trick from the world of ultramarathoning: Do long runs on consecutive days to get a big endurance boost.

As with running twice a day, this idea isn't as crazy as it may sound. If you follow them with a few true recovery days, back-to-back long runs can lead to above-average endurance gains because of super compensation, wherein your body reacts to an extraordinary stimulus by preparing for its recurrence.

A decade ago I was preparing to run Maryland's C&O Canal in a week. To get ready to average a marathon a day for a week, I did regular back-to-back long runs of 20 to 22 miles. After the first couple times, I had adjusted, and the second of the two long runs was no more work than the first. Knowing that I had to go long again the following day kept me from running the first day's run too hard, and it gave me great motivation to do all the little things afterward to optimize recovery. I definitely felt more aerobically strong after a few weekends of consecutive long runs.

Back-to-back long runs work well in traditional training programs in the early to middle phases. For example, if you're training for a marathon and have a few good long runs under your belt, you could do back-to-back long runs two of the weekends in the coming month. Keep the pace nice and gentle on both; just concentrate on getting the distance in. As you get closer to your marathon, you would want to move back to one high-quality long run per week for more specific preparation.

41

When One Run a Day Just Isn't Enough

Most top runners run twice a day most days. This isn't as crazy an undertaking as it might sound.

Running twice a day (a.k.a. doubling) is a simple way to increase your mileage. Just three additional short runs a week will boost your weekly mileage by more than 10.

Here's the potentially counterintuitive thing about doubling: it can be a less taxing way to increase your mileage than making all of your runs longer. At some point, adding to individual runs can mean finishing most of those runs a little too fatigued. That's especially undesirable if your form starts to deteriorate, at which point the pounding of running will take more of a toll. By splitting some days' running into two sessions, you spread that stress over more time and are more likely to have good form throughout the day's mileage. If you're to where you're running an hour or most days, breaking some of those days into two runs will leave you fresher while giving you the same fitness benefits.

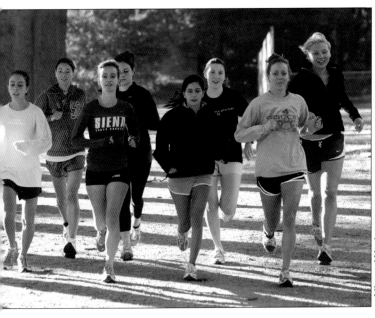

: Alison Wade

42

Handling Double Duty

The first thing to consider about doubling is the time factor. Two runs of 4 and 6 miles will take more total time out of your day than one run of 10 miles, because of the attendant pre- and post-run activities. So if you already struggle to find time for one run a day, forget doubling.

But if you can find the time two or three days a week, experiment to see if doubling works for you. Start by adding a short, very easy run on days when you do your hardest workouts. For example, if you have a group track workout every Tuesday night, do an easy jog of a few miles that morning. Once you adjust to the general concept of doubling, which shouldn't take more than a few weeks, you'll feel better, readier to go fast, on that day's harder session. If your hard workouts are in the morning, then a short, gentle jog that evening will speed your recovery; another round of

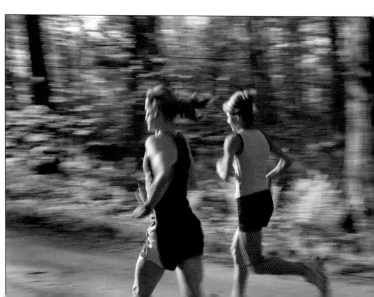

: Stacey Cramp

increased blood flow will bring more nutrients and general looseness to your muscles, sort of like a massage on the go.

Next you could add a second run on one of your standard distance days. Instead of, say, doing one 8-mile run, you could do a 3-miler and 6-miler. It's usually best to keep one of the runs longer than the other on a double day. That helps you to sort of sneak up your mileage totals with less strain while best advancing your fitness.

Add doubles to other days as your enthusiasm and schedule allow. Max out doubling on all other days instead of doubling on your long-run days. After a long run, your priority for the rest of the day is recovering so that you can resume good training as soon as possible. When you've purposefully done a long run to induce muscular fatigue, running again that day will delay getting over that fatigue.

43

Doubles Will Shorten Your Recovery Time

When you first start doubling, expect to feel a little more tired on most runs, especially on double days. But if you add them gradually and wisely, soon you'll notice that you recover quicker from all your runs, even on days you don't double. Your body gets used to running again 6 or 8 hours after a run instead of 24. Your "recoverability," for lack of a better word, improves. In turn, that should allow you to train harder even on days when you don't double—with better recoverability, you can push hard one day and not be as trashed the next day.

44

Doubles on Easy Days?

Twenty years ago, the day after a long run was one of the days of the week I was least likely to double. I slept in, then ran 8 to 10 miles after work. Now that I'm in my midforties, the day after a long run is one of the days I'm most likely to double. Because I'm used to doubling, two runs of 30 to 40 minutes each result in less total fatigue for the day than if I were to run that much all at once.

Similarly, I'm not alone among aging longtime runners in finding that following a hard workout day with a day of a 4- and 8-miler takes less out of me than doing one 10-miler that day. Because of age, there's a greater energy cost associated with that single longer run. For one thing, that 10-miler takes me 10 minutes longer than it used to, so it's more likely that toward the end of the run I'll be fairly fatigued and my form will start to deteriorate. As a result, the day is more likely to make me more tired rather than helping me recover from the previous day's hard work.

You don't have to wait to be my age to get this benefit from doubling. Once you're accustomed to running twice a day, doing so on your recovery days is a great way to make sure they serve their purpose.

45

Final Thought on Running More

Several years ago, a training partner of mine lost some motivation and went from running 70 to 80 miles a week to half that. After a couple years at the lower mileage, he got inspired to return to his former mileage. When he got back to his old mileage, we were out for a run one day when he voiced a great truism: In some ways, he said, it's easier to run more than less.

What he meant is that as you get fitter, each individual run becomes less taxing. As you get fitter, your normal workaday runs feel more like they happen on their own, and you're just along for the ride.

You pass through certain thresholds of fitness as you start running more. What used to be a big deal, maybe a 10-mile run, becomes more like a normal day. The miles just sort of start accumulating on their own. If you run significantly less than usual for even a few days, you start to feel off, you start to lose the overarching rhythm to your running, and your body becomes eager to get back to what has become its higher-mileage set point.

If you've never experienced the feeling of being so fit that it's easier to run more than less, let me assure you it's worth working for.

~⌒

PART TWO

Running Faster:
63 Tips to Help Build Your Speed,
Even If You're Never Going to Race

All other things being equal, pretty much all runners would like to be faster. Wouldn't you? Even if you have no plans to race in the next however long, the thought of being faster than you currently are probably has more appeal than the thought of being slower than you currently are.

Of course, if you do plan to race, then wanting to go faster is a given. You want to know what to do in your daily training to be able to cover a given distance in less time, and you want to know what to do on race day to run as fast as you're capable of that day.

That's what the tips in this chapter are about. We'll look at the main types of workouts that make you faster, as well as how to best build those workouts into your training, how to race to best make use of your fitness, and other things you can do to get faster. We'll also look at some of the mental aspects of running faster. First, though, let's start with why all runners should do regular fast running.

46

First of Two Main Reasons All Runners Should Do Some Faster Running

Regularly running at a variety of paces is what should be considered the norm, not an exception that only runners interested in running as fast as possible should bother with. Like a cook who can master a wide range of dishes and techniques, courses and cuisines, a runner who's comfortable at a variety of paces acquires a broad range of proficiency that makes every run better.

What I'll call multipace training simply makes you a more complete runner. Multipace training gives you greater running-specific muscular strength, moves you through a greater range of motion, fully develops all of the internal processes that underlie running, and optimally prepares you for whatever sort of running challenge you want to take on.

I'm not saying that people who don't train at a variety of paces aren't "real runners," whatever that tired phrase might mean. You can lead a satisfying running life by running exactly the same pace for the same distance every day. But there's a whole other type of fitness available to runners who regularly rotate through several types of workouts. It's a fitness that will make your running more enjoyable regardless of whether you ever plan to test it in a race.

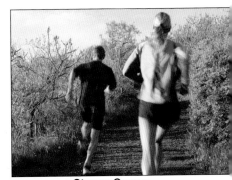

: Stacey Cramp

47

Second of Two Main Reasons All Runners Should Do Some Faster Running

There's no better way to keep your running interesting than to have peaks and valleys of intensity and duration woven throughout your training weeks. Multipace training naturally builds a structure into your running that makes it more enjoyable.

When you regularly do all sorts of workouts, from long runs and basic speed sessions to slow recovery runs and tempo workouts, the variety keeps the days from all blending together. The days have meaning not only in regard to themselves, but to what precedes and follows them. If you've done a long run on Sunday, then you'll probably go slow and short on Monday. That sets you up for a hard workout Tuesday, followed by a recovery day Wednesday. By Thursday maybe a medium-effort run followed by some short, fast quasi-sprints to rev you up for a tempo run on Friday will be the ticket. Then you could finish the week off with an easy day on Saturday to ensure you're good to go long again on Sunday.

To continue our cooking analogy, most people who like to cook find doing so more interesting the more they switch things up, from complex creations to simple stir-fries, from quick scrambles to dishes that take hours to make. In running as in most things in life, not having every day seem like the previous one is motivating.

48
We're All Slower Than Somebody

There's nothing to be gained from belittling yourself over how fast you can run; banish all thoughts of "Oh, I'm so slow, what's the point?" People get lapped even in world-class 10Ks on the track.

There will always be lots of people faster than you. That fact detracts not a whit from your efforts to get faster and the meaning you can find in that pursuit. Any thoughtful runner who has set performance goals and worked hard to reach them will respect any other runner's quest to do the same. Your effort, not your pace at that effort, is what really matters.

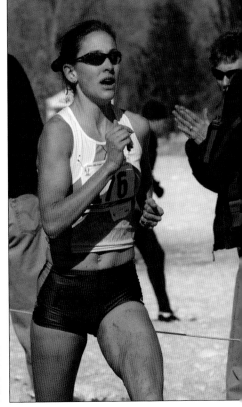

: 101° West

49

Great Training, Not Great Workouts

One more conceptual frame before we look at specific work-outs to get faster: As Pete Magill, the oldest American to break 15:00 for 5K, puts it, there are no great workouts, just great training. Magill means that training is a series of puzzle pieces that link one day's, one week's, one month's efforts to the next. You advance your fitness by gradually building and working steadily toward your goal. Some days that might mean a hard workout, but some days that will mean running very easily to recover from one hard run and prepare for the next.

That's a different, more mature mind-set than the one that says, "I need to go to the track today and run as fast and far as I can to prepare for next week's race." Hard workouts at race pace or faster are necessary to run your best, but they're just one of many building blocks. Focusing on them too much, both physically and mentally, means never reaching your potential.

50

A Crucial Few Types of Fast Running

Potential oversimplification alert: I'm now going to describe some main types of fast workouts. I'm choosing these few types because they're each a targeted way to improve an important aspect of running faster. Nitpickers will say that you can't com-partmentalize running like that; they'll say that all faster running improves several aspects of running fitness. And they're right—you can't say that something like a 3-mile run at the pace you can hold for an hour has only one narrow, easily identified benefit.

At the same time, there are a few key types of workouts that the best runners in the world do over and over again. Each of those workouts are among the most effective ways to improve an important element of running performance. When you understand those few key types of workouts, you can better understand how and why to do them all to become a more complete runner.

51

Improve Your Basic Speed: Striders

All runners should do striders. Yes, all.

By "striders" I mean runs of 100 meters or so, done on flat, level ground after an easy run, at the pace you feel you could hold for a half mile or so. A typical session entails 8 to 12 striders, with as much recovery as you want in between so that you can run the remaining striders with good, relaxed form.

That "relaxed" part is key. Striders are about learning to run fast but free of strain. They're about moving quickly but lightly. Because they're so short, you shouldn't find yourself tying up during them, and your breathing should return to normal soon after.

Striders build your running-specific leg strength and take you through a much greater range of motion than an average easy or moderate run. They'll also help you maintain a light, quick cadence. Striders build a smoother running form, which is then yours to benefit from on all your runs.

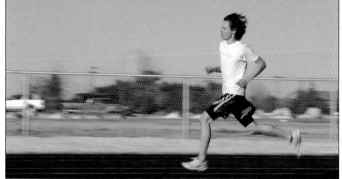

Striders should leave you feeling good, like a kid dashing down the street. American 10K record-holder Chris Solinsky once told me he often does impromptu striders because they're so enjoyable—once you're used to doing them, it's simply fun to run fast.

Do a session of striders once or twice a week, and I guarantee that within a month you'll feel better on most of your runs.

52
A Variation on Striders: Diagonals

Diagonals are a Kenyan specialty that build striders into a slightly more structured workout.

The name comes from the fact that you do them on a rectangular field, like the one inside of a track. You run fast from one corner of the rectangle to the opposite corner, jog along the baseline to the next corner, run fast again across the rectangle to the opposing corner, then jog along the baseline to bring yourself where you started your first fast run. (Imagine an X with lines along the top and bottom of the X; the fast runs cover the lines of the X and the jogs cover the lines along its top and bottom.) As with striders, the fast runs are about 100 meters long. If you're on a rectangular field, the jog between fast runs will take about as long as your fast segments.

Go by time rather than number of fast runs with diagonals. A 10-minute session (counting both fast runs and short jogs) will have you doing about the same number of fast runs as a standard series of striders. If you do 20 or 30 minutes of diagonals, then it's becoming a bit more of a workout that's the focus of your running that day (as opposed to doing a normal run and following it with a quick set of striders). I've done up to 40 minutes of diagonals and can testify that this counts as hard training.

But no matter how long your diagonals session is, running fast but relaxed remains the most important thing. You're still working primarily to improve your basic speed, turnover, and range of motion; those benefits don't come if you allow yourself to get too tired to run the fast parts with good form.

53
Another Variation on Striders: Pick-Ups

Instead of doing an easy run and then doing a series of striders, you can condense things by rolling the striders into the last portion of an easy run.

Say you're out for a 6-miler. With a couple miles to go, you could start alternating 30 seconds at strider pace with 90 seconds of easy running. Repeat that 8 or 10 times and you're home. You could leave things more unstructured by going fast for short stretches as the muse strikes you and jogging to recover until you feel you're ready to run the next pick-up with good form and no strain. This latter approach is better if you're on an undulating course and want to run fast primarily on flat stretches.

54

Improve Your Running Economy: Short Repeats

Moving up from striders and pick-ups, the next main type of faster running is bursts of 60 to 90 seconds at what feels like the pace you could run for a mile. The point of these are to improve your running economy, or how efficient you are (in terms of oxygen consumption) at a given speed. Targeted efforts at this effort level will make you more efficient at all speeds.

Traditionally, this workout is done by doing one-lap repeats of a standard 400-meter track. But there's nothing magical about the distance of 400 meters; it's simply convenient to do one-lap repeats. The important thing here is the amount of time, 60 to 90 seconds, at that intensity of roughly mile race pace. A standard running economy workout would total between 2 and 3 miles worth of hard running, such as ten 400-meter repeats or twelve 300-meter repeats.

These repeats quickly become taxing. So that you can do them all at the right intensity level, you'll need a good recovery jog between. A convenient parameter is to jog for the same distance as your hard bouts. If you're doing the workout based on time, do recovery jogs that last 50 percent to 100 percent as long as your fast runs; for example, 80 seconds hard followed by a 2-minute jog.

55

Improve Your Pumping Ability: VO$_2$ Max Workouts

The next main type of fast running is what are called VO$_2$ max workouts. I'll spare you a lengthy physiology lesson and say simply that these are a targeted way to improve your heart's ability to pump blood and to deliver it efficiently to working muscles.

A typical VO$_2$ max workout consists of runs of 3 to 6 minutes at the pace you could hold for between 2 miles and 5 kilometers; it's convenient to think of them as repeats at 5K race pace. Three to four miles' worth of hard running is a good target, such as six 800-meter repeats or five 1,200-meter repeats. Recovery jogs in VO$_2$ max workouts should last between 50 percent and 100 percent of the time of the repeats. On the track, a one-lap jog between repeats is typical, but for longer repeats like 1 mile, a lap-and-a-half jog is more suitable so that you can run the next repeat at the right pace.

VO$_2$ max workouts are what most people think of if you say you're doing a hard workout. And hard—but effective—they are.

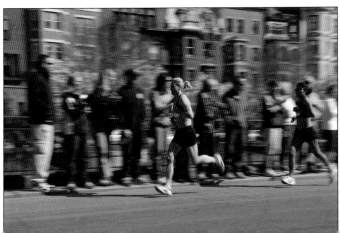

: Stacey Cramp

56

Improve Your Speed Endurance: Short Tempo Runs

There are almost as many definitions of "tempo run" as they are runners. What I mean here are runs of 20 to 30 minutes somewhere between the pace you could hold for an hour to a half marathon. The point of these workouts, often called lactate threshold runs, is to improve your ability to hold a solid pace before having to slow. They do this by making you better at clearing lactate, a by-product of aerobic metabolism that forces you to slow when its presence in your blood becomes too high.

Running for 20 to 30 minutes at the pace you could for an hour to a half marathon is a fairly broad range, and that's fine. The effort level you're after here is what legendary coach Jack Daniels calls "comfortably hard." You're working and have to concentrate to

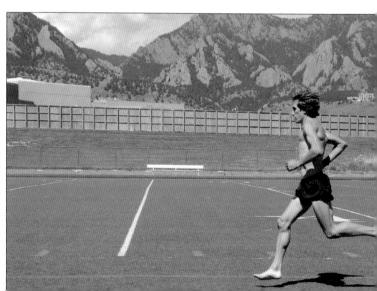

: Brian Metzler

keep the pace going, but you're not under the sort of duress you feel during VO$_2$ max workouts. You should be able to speak in complete sentences on short tempo runs.

Tempo runs are fantastic at building that feeling of solid aerobic strength, where you feel on most runs you can keep going at a strong pace without having to slow. Race performance aside, it's satisfying to know you can do more than run easily for sustained periods. That's why I think even runners with no race plans should do regular tempo runs (and striders!).

57
Improve Your Fatigue Resistance: Long Tempo Runs

The last of the main types of faster running are also known as rhythm runs or marathon-pace runs. The latter name tells you what you need to know about the desired effort level—the fastest pace you could sustain for two to three hours (yes, even if your marathon time is slower than that). These efforts combine some of the benefits of shorter tempo runs with those of long, easy runs. The result is overall improved aerobic strength, in part because of your leg muscles becoming better equipped to receive and make use of the oxygen in your blood.

Long tempo runs can last from 40 to 80 minutes, or 6 to 10 miles if you're thinking in terms of distance. They're typically done as the second part of an otherwise regular long run. But you can also make them their own entity on other days, sandwiching them with a warm-up and cool-down just like you would other types of hard workouts.

58

Hit the Hills

More runners should do hard workouts on hills more regularly. Running hard uphill gives you all the benefits of running hard on flat ground, and then some—greater running-specific leg strength, more muscle fibers recruited (and therefore given an inducement to adapt to a higher work capacity), and of course, specific preparation for tackling hills in races.

Everyone knows intuitively that running fast uphill is hard work, but I don't think that's why ambitious runners avoid hill workouts. After all, they're ambitious runners, so are willing to do almost anything to get faster. I think many people avoid hill workouts because it's not as easy to quantify your workouts on them. If you do a series of 800-meter repeats on a track, you know exactly how "good" of a workout you had, in terms of how your times matched what you were aiming for and what you've done on similar workouts in the recent past. Hill workouts aren't as easily comparable. Even if you always do the same workout on the same stretch of hill, how do you know how that workout compares to an equivalent session on the track? And what about the fact that you may be running hard, but not particularly fast, given the grade?

As a result, runners who might be a little insecure and in need of constant data-driven feedback on their fitness tend to shy away from hill workouts. And that's a shame, because there are several types of hill workouts that are highly effective at making you faster.

59
Good Uphill Running Form

When you're running hard uphill, it's easy to focus so hard on getting to the top that you neglect good running form. Stay mindful of your mechanics on hard uphill runs (and easier ones, for that matter). You may have heard, "Lean into the hill." That's not handy advice if it means you bend forward at the waist; doing that will mean you're fighting gravity even more than the hill is already causing you to.

Maintain a tall running posture, with your chest up, not moving toward your knees. Concentrate on keeping a slight curve in your lower back and your hips forward. My college coach always gave the "pecker out" cue for how to hold our midsection. (He apparently never coached women.) Keep your shoulders low and relaxed. Imagine your hands pulling up a rope that's secured at the top of the hill. A quicker, lighter foot strike will get you to the top faster than purposefully reaching for more ground.

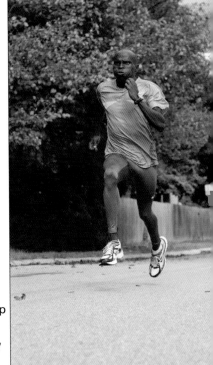

: Stacey Cramp

57

60

Hill Sprints

Hill sprints are like striders in that they'll improve your running form and basic speed. They're also like striders in that they're short enough that you can do them on otherwise easy days and they'll leave you feeling more, not less, ready to run hard the next day.

Hill sprints are runs of only 10 to 15 seconds up the steepest hill you can find. On each one, you should attack the hill "with the mentality of a sprinter," the great Italian coach Renato Canova once explained to me. In other words, all out, as fast as you can. Hill sprints are done "without care for recovery" in Canova's words; that is, recover completely before doing the next one. Walk down the hill, and then walk around some more at the base until you're ready to run the next one "with the mentality of a sprinter." The world-class marathoners Canova coaches take 2 to 3 minutes between their hill sprints.

These are basically like doing squats using your weight and the hill instead of a barbell. Hill sprints strengthen all your running-specific leg muscles, improve your explosive power, and train your legs to recruit more fibers as they tire. That's all good stuff!

The first time you do hill sprints, do just a few, especially if you haven't truly sprinted for awhile. Add one or two per session until you're at 10. There's no reason to do more than that, because you'll be unable to reach the proper intensity. Hill sprints can take the place of striders in your schedule. Once you're used to them, you can do them the day before a hard workout, because they'll prepare your central nervous system to work harder the next day.

61

Short Hills

Fairly steep hills that take you between 30 and 60 seconds to get up can also replace striders as a way to improve your basic speed. These are a staple of Kenyans' training; everyone from milers to marathoners do, say, 15 repeats up a 30-second hill. It's OK on these workouts to not be fully recovered between repeats so that you can also get cardiovascular benefits from the session. As always, though, you want to be getting up the hill with quick, efficient form, and that's not going to possible if you run the first few all-out.

62

Medium Hills

Hills that take about 90 seconds to climb are great for running economy workouts. The grade should be less than for hill sprints and short hills. Your effort should be at about mile race pace; 8 to 10 reps is a good target. Because you're now climbing a fairly lengthy hill, the jog down should give you plenty of time to recover. If, however, you get to the bottom and aren't yet ready to go hard again, jog around a bit more. Hitting the proper intensity is much more important than simply being out of breath the whole time.

63

Long Hills

Hills that take two to four minutes to climb can serve many of the purposes of VO_2 max workouts. And of course if you're preparing for a long race with several hills, like the Boston Marathon, you'll want to be used to sustained uphill efforts.

: 101° West

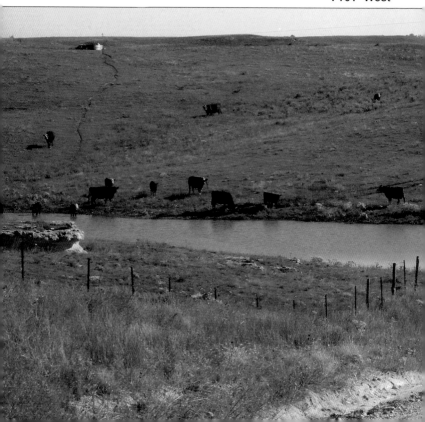

The tricky thing with hills this long is the jog down. First, you'll probably be fully recovered by the time you get to the bottom. That's fine, but you need to be sure you're running the uphill part hard enough to keep your heart rate elevated high enough throughout the workout. Second, there's the issue of pounding—jogging down a half-mile hill six times when you're tired can put a lot of strain on your legs. Stay mindful of your form as you jog down so that you're not crashing into the ground with every step.

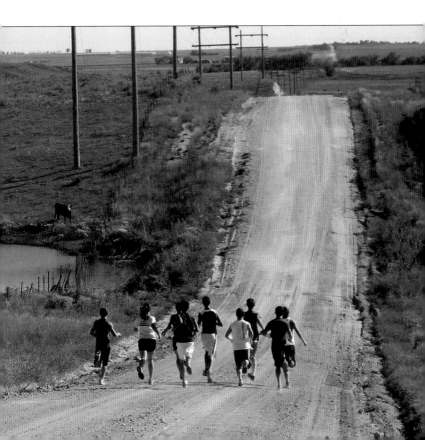

64
Treadmill Hills

Here's one place where a treadmill can be better than "real" running. You can simulate any hill workout on a treadmill without having to deal with potential problems from the repeated jogs down. Just don't set the incline so high that you go flying off the back!

65
Going Downhill Fast

If you want help building your basic speed, why not enlist gravity? Doing striders on a slight downhill can enhance all the benefits of doing them on flat ground, especially your ability to maintain a relaxed, quick cadence at high speed.

The key is to do downhill striders on a relatively gentle descending grade. If it's too steep, your form will be too different from how you run on flat or slightly uphill stretches. A 1 percent or 2 percent grade is good.

As on regular striders, focus on running fast but relaxed. Hold back a bit on the first couple to make sure you're adequately warmed up, and then let 'er rip—on the last several of a set of 10 striders, see how fast of a turnover you can maintain without your form deteriorating. Walk or jog gently up the hill in between. After a month of weekly downhill striders, you should notice improvements in your form on your hard workouts and in your speed at the end of races.

66

The Mental Side of Running Fast

Let's not neglect the mental benefits that regular fast running bring to the rest of your running. Pushing yourself as you do on hard workouts will help you learn how to dole out your mental capital on other runs and will show you that you can usually keep going even when the urge to quit or slow significantly is overwhelming. Tempo runs are especially good at developing your ability to mentally see things through and wait out physical sensations that are more wearing than acutely painful.

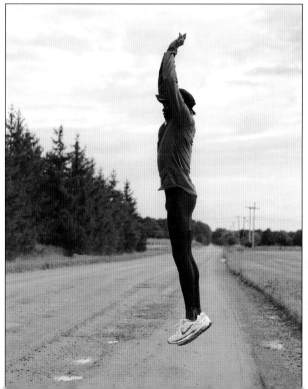

: Stacey Cramp

67
Relax, Relax, Relax

Watch the best runners in the world race, and you'll notice that almost all of them look supremely relaxed at almost all times. The grimacers and grunters and strainers are the exceptions (and usually the ones finishing behind). Sprinters are especially adept at running relaxed and letting the speed come out.

It might be natural to think that because you're working harder you should feel tenser. But it's not helpful. Straining while you run causes unnecessary muscle tightness and fatigue, and wastes energy that could better be used on getting to the finish line faster.

Everyone can get better at running fast but relaxed through practice. On your harder workouts, frequently run through a mental checklist: Are my shoulders low and even? Are my hands cupped loosely? Is my face, especially my jaw, free of strain?

Doing striders is an excellent opportunity to consciously work on running fast but relaxed. On each strider, think about one element of a flowing, relaxed running gait. Over time, practicing these desirable movement patterns will come naturally, even when you're under duress in the last third of a race.

68
Group Benefits

If there's ever a time to seek the company of other runners, it's for your hard workouts. Even paragons of mental toughness find they more often meet their hard-session goals by doing the workouts with one or more partners.

In addition to helping you get through the session mentally, workout partners can help you practice race tactics, such as tucking in behind someone else and drawing off her energy. You also get the physical benefit of others breaking the wind if you have different people lead different parts of the workout.

Doing workouts with others can also help you run more within yourself if you tend to push too hard in most hard sessions. Which leads us to . . .

69

It's a Workout, Not a Race

The purpose of any workout, even the hardest, is to advance your fitness toward a performance goal. That means a measured effort that's hard enough to provide the desired stimulus, but not so hard that you're so trashed that the next few days of run-

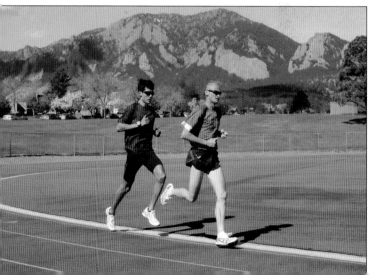

: Brian Metzler

ning are a waste. Remember Pete Magill's counsel: great training, not great workouts. Elite runners go to the well seldom if ever in their training; they save their racing for the races.

You should finish hard workouts with more in the tank. If you're doing repeats, you should be able to run a few more at the same pace. If you're doing a tempo run, you should be able to run another couple miles at the same pace without a marked increase in effort.

70
Scheduling Fast Workouts

A good training program regularly includes all of the above main types of workouts. Blending them together ensures that you've developed in a targeted way the key components of sustained fast running. If you're really focusing on a particular race distance, you'd want to give one type of training more emphasis (such as tempo runs if you're pointing toward a half marathon), but you should still do all the other workouts regularly. If you're aiming more for general race fitness to be able to compete well at a variety of common distances, then rotating through them all regularly is perfect preparation.

An ambitious runner during a non-race week would typically aim for a longer and shorter fast workout, plus a long run and a day with some work on basic speed (striders, pick-ups, hill sprints, short hills, etc.). In planning your hard training, think more in blocks of a month than a week. Planning in seven-day cycles can lead you to try to cram too much in every week and skimp on your recovery days, rather than do the hard work and see how you recover.

Over a month, you can more realistically and fruitfully plan where to place the key elements of multipace training. If in a month you can do three good long runs, two tempo runs, two VO_2 max workouts, two running economy workouts, and four basic speed sessions, you're doing great. And you'll probably be able to repeat that level of quality the next month, and the month after that. Long periods of training a little less hard than you could are much better long-term than occasional killer weeks interspersed with significantly more modest training.

71

If You Feel Good, Go

"Don't waste good time" was the advice of Kenyan John Ngugi, who won an Olympic 5K and five world cross-country titles. He meant that you needn't feel constrained by a written training schedule. If you plan to run hard on Wednesday but find yourself champing at the bit while running Tuesday, go, get in a hard run then. If you were to wait until the next day, you might not feel anywhere near as full of running.

Ngugi was in his twenties when he said "don't waste good time," but his advice is especially useful for older runners. With age, the day-to-day changes in energy level become more varied and unpredictable. If you happen upon an unexpected feeling of vibrancy, take advantage of it. Many of my tempo runs these days come about by heeding Ngugi's advice—I'll be 2 miles into a run and decide it's the right time to run hard for the next 20 or 30 minutes.

The only day not to take this tack is the day after a hard workout. Err on the side of caution on those days, no matter how incredible you feel, by keeping the pace gentle.

72

A Workout Variation: Ladders

Instead of doing a workout where all your repeats are the same distance, do ladders, where you start short, get longer, and then come back down. A typical ladder when doing repeats at 5K race pace would be repeats of one 400-meter lap, then two laps, on up to four laps, before coming back down one lap at a time to finish with a 400-meter repeat. Ladders are a good way to ease into a workout physically and mentally. On the way back down, you could run the last couple repeats a bit faster to practice picking up the pace while already very tired.

A potential drawback to ladders is that they get mentally easier once you're coming back down. In races, of course, there's no such easing of the mental strain as the finish approaches.

73

Another Variation: Fast Finishes

Finish some of your longer repeat workouts, like miles or kilometers, with a few 200s or 300s. You'll be pleasantly surprised at how fast you can run the short segments once you're fully warmed up. I once set a 200-meter PR on the last of four 200s done impromptu after a set of six 800s.

74

Yet Another Variation: Fartlek

When most people talk about fartlek workouts, they're really talking about doing a structured workout, like ten 2-minute repeats with a 2-minute recovery jog, elsewhere than the track. True fartlek is in the spirit of its translation from the Swedish, "speed play," and isn't structured. You go hard for as long as you feel like it, recover for as long as you want, go hard again, perhaps for a different distance at a different pace, jog until you feel ready to go again, and stop the workout when you feel like you've done enough hard running for the day.

Fartleks are great for runners who need to get better at accurately judging how to dole out their hard efforts. They'll teach you how to sense when you're ready to push and when you need to back off. They're also a needed counterweight to the tendency too many runners have to judge their fitness solely by the readings on their watches.

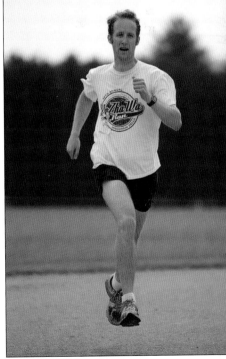

: Alison Wade

75
"Half" Workouts

Not every "hard" workout has to be a killer session. You can sneak in more quality without going to the well by stopping by a track or hill or obstacle-free stretch of road toward the end of a run and doing a few up-tempo repeats of between 200 and 800 meters.

76
Current vs. Goal Pace

Do almost all of your fast running at your current race paces, not your goal race paces. That will ensure that you're running within yourself and working at the proper intensity, rather than straining to run times that might have no relation to your fitness. After all, if it really worked to pick an arbitrary time and start training at that race pace and inevitably run that race time, well, then excuse me while I go start doing all my hard workouts at sub-4:00 mile pace.

First, do the training at your current capabilities. That will advance your fitness. That will lead to faster race times. Adjust your workout times only after you've run the faster races that justify them.

77
Paces in Perspective

When you hear people faster than you talk about their training, translate their workouts into efforts relative to race pace. A 20-miler with the last 8 miles at 5:00 per mile sounds really fast—and it is—but for an elite man, it's a long run with the last portion at marathon race pace. That's the sort of workout most people prepping for a marathon can and should do.

Focus on the general patterns and effort levels in others' training, not the precise numbers that happen to coincide with those effort levels for a given person.

78

Where to Run Fast

We tend to think of hard workouts in terms of repeats of a 400-meter track. Certainly tracks provide objective data on how fast you run for how far, and that data is easy to compare to how you did last week or last month for the same workout.

But doing the bulk of your hard workouts on a track can be a crutch. It's easy to get used to getting split times every 400 meters, or even 200 meters, and then adjusting the pace if necessary. But most of us run most of our races on the roads. When was the last time you got 400-meter splits in a road race? Doing too many workouts on the track and judging your success by how well you hit your splits means you don't develop as good a sense of judging your effort using your body's feedback. Yet your body's feedback is mostly what you're going to rely on in your races: Am I going out too fast? Starting too slow? Can I push it a bit more on this hill? Can I hold this effort to the finish?

A good compromise if you're starting a training cycle is to do your first few hard workouts on a track to get a sense of what your basic paces feel like. Then do most of your hard workouts by time away from the track; for example, instead of six 800-meter repeats with a one-lap recovery jog, do six hard 3-minute runs at 5K race effort with a 2-minute recovery jog. You can easily translate all the main types of hard workouts into minutes instead of distance.

79
Horses for Courses

Another reason to do many of your hard workouts away from the artificial setting of a track is to practice running hard on the types of courses you'll race on. Hard sessions and tempo runs on roads mean you'll be running on flats and around corners and up and down hills and all the other elements you'll encounter in a typical road race. You'll also better prepare your muscles and tendons for handling the increased pounding that accompanies fast running on asphalt.

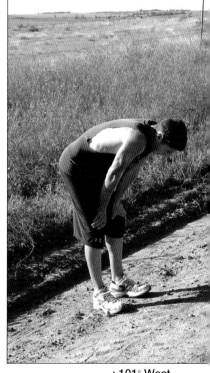

: 101° West

80

When a Workout Isn't Going Well

There will be tough days at the office. As with triage on a non-great long run, how to proceed depends on what's happening.

If you're not hitting your goal times because of an acute running-related pain, stop. Trying to run fast is going to make the nascent injury worse.

If your times are off because of the weather, carry on. Accept that your times are going to be slower than you want and focus on getting in the right effort.

If your times are slightly off for no obvious reason, carry on. You don't want to get in the habit of cutting a workout short simply because it's not going as well as you think it should.

If your times are significantly off from what you've recently run in similar workouts, then you should probably pull the plug on the workout. By "significantly off" I mean "what the hey is going on?" off, like a difference of 5 seconds a lap. You're either carrying too much residual fatigue from your running or the rest of your life to put forth the right effort, or you're on the verge of getting sick. You need to rest up until you're ready to handle hard training again.

81

More Support for Off-Track Running

Notice that all the above scenarios stem from a track setting. Here's another reason to do many of your hard workouts by time and effort away from the track: You don't have to have these conversations with yourself. If your workout is six 3-minute repeats at 5K effort on the roads, then there are fewer ways to tell yourself, "This isn't going well." You simply get in the effort at whatever pace turns out to be appropriate that day for the combination of your energy level and environment.

82
What's a Good Warm-Up?

The need to prepare your body for fast running is intuitive. What might not be so obvious is what makes a good warm-up. A jog of 1.5 to 3 miles is the first step, but not the only step. On the jog, start slower than you usually do on typical runs. This is really the day to gradually bring your body to life. By the end of your warm-up jog, you should be moving fluidly and faster than you were at the beginning without any real increase in effort.

Follow your warm-up jog with some dynamic stretches, like leg swings and skipping. Right before fast running, these are better than static stretching at preparing your muscles to work hard. Then do 4 to 8 striders of 80 to 100 meters, building into running faster on each one. Don't worry that this fast running will detract from your workout; it will better prepare you to do the first couple repeats at the right intensity with the right range of motion.

If your workout is repeats of 2 minutes or more, after your last strider, run for 30 to 60 seconds at the pace you want to hit on the first repeat; on the track, running for 200 meters at that pace is convenient. This longer bout will prepare your internal plumbing systems to work at a high rate starting on the first repeat. Take a couple minutes of active rest (walking, more dynamic stretching) between this run and the first repeat of your workout.

83
What's a Good Cool-Down?

The reason to do something other than plop yourself down under a tree after a hard workout might not be as obvious as the rationale for warming up. But cool-downs are important.

To see why, think of a graphical representation of a workout. You move from being sedentary to light activity to harder activity to a peak of activity—the meat of the workout, like 800-meter repeats. At that peak, your body's internal processes are working at a high rate. A good cool-down brings them back down to their normal state gradually, and your body thanks you by being better able to handle the next days of running.

To gradually bring your body down from the metabolic peak it reached during your workout, jog 1 to 3 miles. Follow that with gentle stretching, either dynamic or static, to encourage continued blood flow to the muscles that were recently working hard. This will help to continue to remove waste products and reoxygenate the muscle tissues.

84
Post-Workout Nutrition

After a hard workout, it's typical to not feel like eating for a long time. Nonetheless, you should take in some carbohydrate-rich calories as soon as possible after. After your hardest workouts, your immune system will be suppressed for a few hours; taking in carbs then will undo some of that suppression, and thereby lessen the chance of finding yourself with a cold two days later.

If your stomach is so unsettled after a hard workout that solid food is a no-go, have a couple hundred calories' worth of sport drink within the first hour of finishing.

85

Get Faster Without Running Fast

Running form drills can help you run faster by eliminating weakness and hitches in your gait. Each drill focuses on one aspect of good running form, such as a good back-kick or high knees, so that moving in that way becomes more natural to you. Over time, the improved movement patterns become ingrained in your normal running stride, and you can run faster with less risk of injury.

Start incorporating running form drills into your routine by doing them once a week after an easy run. Doing them the same day you do striders is an excellent choice. Once you become used to doing the drills, do some as part of your warm-up before hard workouts; in that setting, they'll help you be ready to run the first repeat with good, fluid form.

Elite coaches Greg McMillan and Jay Johnson have each produced excellent DVDs on running form drills. The DVDs demonstrate the proper form for each drill so that you can get the greatest benefit from your work.

86

How's Your Turnover?

The number of times your feet hit the ground per minute is partly fixed by genetics and the standard operation of your central nervous system. There's no perfect cadence for distance running, but you'll run faster with more efficiency and less strain if you get your turnover up to at least 170 foot strikes per minute. (Determine this by counting the number of times one foot hits the ground in a minute, and doubling.)

If your turnover is less than 170, make a conscious effort on some runs to cover the ground with a quicker cadence. Striders at least once a week are crucial to bumping up your natural stride rate. You can also do a fast feet shuffle after some runs to train your central nervous system to work more rapidly. Without really lifting your feet, shuffle along as quickly as you can for 10 seconds. Walk around for a minute, and repeat twice.

: Alison Wade

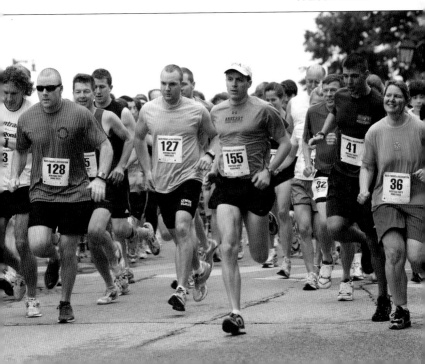

87

Shoes for Running Fast

If you're going to race, get racing shoes. Less weight on your feet lowers your oxygen cost at a given pace, which should translate to racing faster.

The problem people run into with racing shoes is muscular fatigue and soreness, during and after races, usually in the calf and Achilles areas. That's a consequence of the shoes typically having lower heels and less cushioning than training shoes. Easy solution: wear your racing shoes for your hard workouts. Doing so prepares your muscles and tendons for the slighter shoes on race day. Wearing your racing shoes in training can also help you run those hard workouts faster and with the lighter, more efficient form you want when running faster.

88

What Does Running Slow Have to Do with Running Fast?

Remember good old tip number 77, about translating faster runners' workout paces to race pace to put them in perspective? It's also helpful to understand elites' recovery paces relative to race paces. A national-class woman who runs easy mileage at 7:30 per mile is doing those recovery runs more than 2 minutes per mile slower than her 10K race pace. Do you?

Probably not. One of the greatest differences I've observed in how elites and other runners train pertains to recovery days. Elites place as much importance on the right effort level the day after a hard workout as they do on the right effort level the day of a hard workout. They know that it's on those recovery days that their bodies produce the adaptations to the stimulus of hard running that results in greater fitness. Allowing that adaptation to occur via a day of really easy running means they get the most out of their hard work. And why wouldn't you want to get the maximum benefits from your hard work?

89
The Best Use of a Heart Rate Monitor

With just a little experience at regular fast running, you can tell from your internal sensory data if you're working at the right intensity. So while heart rate monitors can provide additional support to your feeling that, yes, this is an effort level I could sustain for an hour, they're not necessary on those runs for most people.

Instead, the best use of a heart rate monitor for most runners is to make sure you're not going too fast on your recovery days. When you're used to plugging away at about the same effort level most days, consciously keeping things below 70 percent of your maximum heart rate can feel absurdly slow. But that seemingly too-gentle level of effort is what you need after a hard workout to truly recover. If you have the common struggle of running your easy days too fast, set a heart rate monitor to beep if you go above 70 percent of max. If it beeps, slow down until the beeping stops.

90

Determining Your Max Heart Rate

For a heart rate monitor to help you, you need to know your max heart rate. All the standard formulas, like 220 minus your age, are rubbish; they're based on averages that have no applicability to you as an individual.

To get a reasonably close reading of your max, wear your heart rate monitor on a few VO_2 max workouts. The highest reading you get toward the end of the workout should be within a few beats of your max heart rate. You can also get good data from a workout of ten really fast 2-minute uphill runs or a 5K race.

91

Important Concept for Race Preparation

Getting race-fit isn't like cramming for a test. A sudden slew of hard workouts in the two weeks before a race are a lot more likely to leave you overly fatigued and injured rather than significantly fitter. The important work happens more steadily, less dramatically in the months before an important race.

If you're heading into a race feeling unprepared, avoid crash training. Revise your goal for the race, run it such that you draw some positives from it and review what went wrong in your build-up so that you can be better prepared the next time.

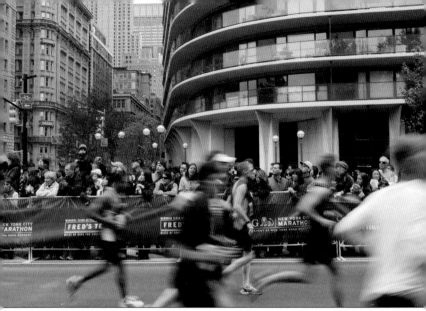

: Stacey Cramp

92

A Meaningful Mantra Regardless of Race Distance

In the first half of the race, don't be an idiot. In the second half of the race, don't be a wimp.

93

Ignore Others the First Third of the Race

The main cause of people not racing to their potential is starting too fast. Even runners who have sworn to run even pace from the gun lose their heads in that first mad dash off the line. They get sucked into starting too fast, in part because the people they want to beat seem so far ahead.

Ignore the madding crowd in the first third of races. You're not obligated to run lemming-like and follow others who are botching their performances by starting too fast. If you want to beat specific people, the way to do that is to be ahead of them at the finish line, not the 1-mile mark. Running the fastest time you're capable of on that day will almost always mean running the same pace throughout the race. Do that, and you'll catch the too-fast starters by the last third of the race. As you pass them, they'll be unable to respond because they'll be too busy paying for their early-race brashness.

94

Race Pointer: 5K

Starting too fast is exceedingly common in 5Ks. Unfortunately, among common distances, it's the one where you can least afford to misjudge pace in the first mile. The race is so short and you're running so close to your aerobic capacity that there's not time to recover and regroup from an early pacing mistake. Instead, if you start too fast, somewhere in the second mile you'll get a sense of impending doom. A few minutes later, your breathing will go into overdrive, and you'll be forced to slow. Whatever time cushion you built with a fast opening mile will disappear, and then some, as you struggle to the finish.

Regular workouts at 5K pace should teach you the right effort in the first mile. Doing some of those workouts on uncalibrated courses will better teach you what the right effort level should feel like. Even if you do all of your 5K pace workouts on the track, use the workouts as a way to learn the proper effort level for the first mile of 5K races. During track workouts, look at your watch only at the end of a repeat; adjust your effort accordingly on the next repeat if you're too fast or too slow. That will better prepare you than checking your workout splits every half a lap. You won't get those splits in a race when you would most benefit from them.

95
Race Pointer: 10K

One key to running your best 10K is to not run the first mile at 5K pace. For most runners, that's a difference of only 10 to 15 seconds per mile. But that's a significant difference in effort level. If you're already breathing every second step in the second mile of a 10K, you've gone out too fast. To keep the race from becoming a complete disaster, back off for a few minutes to allow your breathing to slow, then pick up the pace again.

96
Race Pointer: 15K to Half Marathon

Mental lapses are common in the middle of races like 15K, 10 miles, 20K, and half marathon. If you're really racing the distance, like a minute or more per mile than your normal training pace, you need to concentrate the whole time. The proper pace shouldn't feel all that hard in terms of your breathing for most of the race, but you'll still have to bear down to keep the proper effort going. Otherwise, it's common for your mile splits to start being 10 or 15 seconds slower.

The benefit from tempo runs of learning how to keep that concentration going can't be overstated.

97

Race Pointer: Marathon

Expend as little mental energy as possible in the first 15 miles of a marathon. That doesn't mean to disregard your pace or be nonchalant about taking drinks or not monitoring how you're feeling. It means that if you're too engaged mentally, like responding to every move made by runners around you, then you're too caught up in it too early. You're not going to be able to hold that level of exertion, both physical and mental, until the end. Anyone who has crashed over the last miles of a marathon, me included, will tell you it's an experience worth avoiding.

If you're properly trained, the pace in the first half of a marathon should take care of itself; as much as possible, put your body and mind on autopilot. If you have the common experience of the pace feeling so easy that you go faster than goal pace without trying, restrain yourself. Running at that slightly faster pace is burning extra fuel you'll need every ounce of after the 20-mile mark. Save the pace pushing and heroics for the last 10K.

98

What's a Good Race Warm-Up?

Except for marathons, where you don't need much more than some easy jogging and stretching, use your standard hard workout warm-up for races. Time things so that you finish your striders about 10 minutes before the start. Then do this: Run for 60 to 90 seconds at your tempo run pace. Finish this run about five minutes before the start; jog and move lightly as needed and possible to stay loose.

That little burst at tempo pace will prepare your body to work at a higher metabolic level, which will mean that launching into race pace won't be such a shock. This little trick picks up on the observation most runners make that the second repeat of a hard workout often feels much easier than the first one.

If you're properly trained, you should have no concern that warming up fairly aggressively will detract from your race performance.

99

Not Every Race Is the Olympics

Don't expect to reach peak performance in every race. Comparing every race to your personal best for the distance is unrealistic. Most races are building blocks to later, faster performances, not ultimate ends in themselves. If you ran up to your potential on the day, considering factors like your recent training, the course, the weather, and your mental fortitude, what more can you ask of yourself?

100
Races as Workouts

"The best workout is a race," goes the old saying. Using races to break up the monotony of training is an excellent idea and a good way to overcome thinking about every race the be-all and end-all of your running. If you get nervous before important races, using races as workouts gives you more practice at going through race-day logistics calmly.

There are lots of options here: Jump in a 5K as a tempo run. Experiment with finishing fast by running the first half of a 10K at tempo pace, then picking up the pace over the second half. Use a 10-miler or half marathon as a venue for a marathon-pace run where you can practice taking fluids at race pace and running in a large pack.

101
State Your Race Goals

Before a race, be able to articulate three goals: First, the ultimate outcome of the day. (Again, this shouldn't always be to set a personal record.) Second, a specific answer to "What are the main things you want to achieve in this race?" Third, if things don't go as well as hoped, one or two things you'll be able to salvage to come out with a positive experience.

102

Tapering Your Training

When cutting back your training before important races, keep some quality. Going from regular multipace training to nothing but easy runs will leave you feeling flat come race day.

A really hard workout the week of an important race won't improve your fitness in time for race day, so there's no point in risking lingering fatigue from it. Try something like 400- or 600-meter repeats at race pace five days before a key race as a way to further ingrain what that pace feels like into your muscle memory. Two days before the race, do a session of striders to keep your central nervous system revved up and your running form working through its full range of motion.

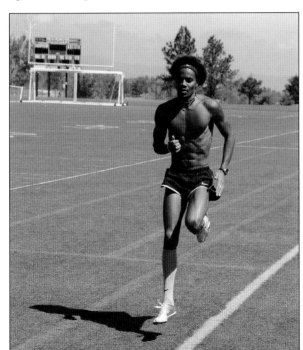

: BrianMetzler

103
Race Distance ≠ Your Worth as a Runner

With the increased popularity of the half marathon and marathon in recent years, it's become more common to equate one's race distance with one's "seriousness" as a runner. This is nonsense. The best milers in the world regularly do 100-mile weeks to prepare for a race they'll finish in less than four minutes. Never let anyone question your running credentials simply because you choose to see how fast you can go for in shorter races.

104
About Those Early Race Starts

Most road races start early in the morning to avoid heat and traffic complications. If you do most of your hard workouts in the afternoon or evening, it's worth shifting an occasional one to the morning so that you have some practice at running fast so early. Most of the bodily functions involved in fast running peak in the late afternoon, so you need to teach your body how to function at a high level at what it considers an inconvenient time.

Early-morning workouts once a month will also give you a chance to experiment with matters such as how soon before running hard you should get up and what your stomach can tolerate then.

105

Maintenance Mode

Most of us will have periods where real life intrudes and we're unable to train as desired. (For example, let's say you're finishing writing a book while working a full-time job.) Keep some quality in your training when you know there will be interruptions for a week to a month. You can emerge from such a period without significant losses in fitness by maintaining the basic structure of multipace training.

If your jammed period means you can still run every day but have less time on those days, do mini versions of your usual hard sessions. For example, instead of a good warm-up, a long tempo run, and a solid cool-down, you could head out on a 5-mile loop. Use the first mile as your warm-up, run hard for 3 miles, and jog home as your cool-down. Similarly, do six 30-second pick-ups toward the end of a run instead of a full-blown set of striders after the run.

If your busy time means you have fewer days per week to run, keep at least one day of striders and one day of a longer workout. If you feel too stressed out to do one of your standard sessions, this is a perfect opportunity for a more unstructured fartlek workout, where you run fast and easy as the spirit moves you.

106

Feel Better by Running Faster

When you're feeling flat, a little fast running is often the best cure. A slow 5 miles might leave you feeling more lethargic. Instead, throw in some random short pick-ups, or do a set of striders on your street once you've done your normal loop. Because they get your central nervous system working at a higher level but aren't long enough to wear you down, little bursts of fast running can help you surpass sluggishness.

107

Sorry, but Speed Is a Use-It-or-Lose-It Phenomenon

Always stay in touch with your basic speed. You'll spend a lot more time just getting back to where you were if you ignore it for weeks at a time than you will tending to it once or twice a week throughout the year. You don't need to do hands-on-knees sets of 200s every week to maintain your speed. Fast, relaxed striders toward the end of an easy run or immediately following one will go a long way toward preserving your turnover and the increased range of motion that comes only with running near top-end speed.

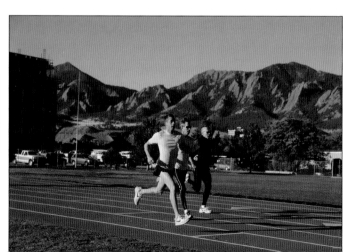

: Brian Metzler

108

Final Thought on Running Faster

Elite runners are born with great physical gifts that become obvious once they start training hard. But they really reach their potential by having a mind-set that all of us, regardless of our genetics, can adopt.

How many times have you had a good string of training going, but then have a bad workout, and suddenly freak out about what kind of shape you're in? How often has one sub-par race come to be taken as the new norm of your fitness?

The elites who consistently achieve excellence think otherwise. I've talked with scores of national- and world-class runners whose outlook I've come to think of as "reality-based optimism." That is, they have confidence that great things will happen if they do the right work. They see a fabulous workout or race as a hint of what they can achieve, not a unique occurrence.

In contrast, a couple of bad workouts, or a worse-than-expected race, are taken as aberrations. They're indications that something is amiss, and are opportunities for analysis: Am I not sleeping enough? Did I run like an idiot? Were my expectations in line with my current fitness? Am I on the verge of being sick? And so on.

Have faith that, if your training is correct and your goals are realistic but challenging, you can surpass your current performance level. Be excited by a good workout or race—that's an indication that you're heading in the right direction. Realize that a bad workout or race happens for a reason. Instead of thinking that it's a true indication of your fitness, determine why your performance was off, and then figure out how to prevent it from recurring.

PART THREE

Running Injury-Free: 50 Tips to Help You Avoid, Treat, and Beat Injuries

No runner wants to get injured.

When you're hurt, what's normally one of the highlights of your day becomes an opportunity for endless rumination and worry; what's usually a source of stress relief becomes a source of stress. When you're hurt, you become achingly familiar with the famous five stages of grief—denial, anger, bargaining, depression, acceptance—in part because you can go through all five within the space of a 30-minute run. When you're hurt, things just don't seem right with the world. So let's agree that not getting injured should be one of your major, ongoing, underlying goals, whether you're a miler or marathoner, a new runner or a lifetimer, a weekly racer or someone who has no interest in ever stepping to a start line.

Unfortunately, injuries are a fact of running life. Moreover, you don't have to have a full-blown can't-run-down-the-street-without-falling-over injury for something to be irksome enough that it interferes with your running. In fact, in some ways, chronic little niggles that you can run through can be more frustrating than major injuries, because they leave you in a constant guessing game, and it's easy to accept them as a given, despite the toll they take on your running.

The tips in this chapter stem from a three-part way of thinking about running injuries. The first I've already stated—being injured stinks, so let's try to avoid it. Second, when you're injured or have a chronic low-level pain associated with running, you need to do things to get the immediate situation under control. What those things are varies among injuries. Third, all injuries are evidence of some underlying problem with your running body. An injury is an opportunity to investigate what that root problem might be, and then devise a plan for addressing it long-term so that the injury doesn't recur.

Let's start, then, by looking in general at why you get injured, how to know if you should keep running on your injury, and when to seek professional help. Then we'll look at some immediate treatments for common running injuries, as well as ways to maintain your fitness when you're injured. Finally, I'll share some thoughts on the most effective ways to build a running body that's highly resistant to injury so that you can better pursue your running at the level you want to.

109
What's a Running Injury?

Almost all running injuries are overuse injuries rather than acute injuries. That is, they're caused by one or more body parts being unable over time to hold up to the repetitive stress of running, rather than a sudden, dramatic insult to the body, like a basketball player tearing her Achilles tendon or a football player destroying his ACL. The good news stemming from this fact is that almost all running injuries are short-term conditions. If you intervene early enough, you can calm the protesting body part and encourage it along the path back to cooperating when you run.

It's often said that injuries are caused by runners trying to run too far, too fast, or both. While that's true in one sense—you probably wouldn't develop that strained calf or sore hamstring if you never ran—it's a bit of a simplistic view. What's easy for your knee to handle when it's warm and you're on vacation and running on a flat dirt path might be too much it's cold and you've been working like crazy (probably sitting a lot) and you're running in the dark on the edge of a slanted asphalt road. Always be mindful of the entire context in which your running occurs, both to avoid injuries and to figure out causes if one occurs.

110

A Medical Model

A helpful framing method is to think about injury the way you might think about diseases with strong lifestyle risk factors—there are genetic components, but much of what happens is under your control. Someone trying to lower her risk for coronary artery disease would make certain choices, such as eating a diet low in saturated fat, not smoking, exercising regularly, and maintaining a good weight. Similarly, you can strongly control the risk factors for running injury through such choices as maintaining a good balance between hard and easy efforts, running on level, soft surfaces when possible, maintaining good muscle and joint strength and flexibility, ditching broken-down running shoes, and so on.

111
Beware of Modern Life!

Related to that last thought: Modern life should be considered a risk factor for running injuries. Driving for hours at a time, sitting slumped over a laptop, cocking your head to one side while on the phone, seldom moving through all planes of motion—these common ways of spending our days can set you up for injury by tightening and weakening your major muscle groups and throwing your body out of whack. One muscle therapist I know eventually figured out that a teen runner's sudden cycle of injury stemmed from her texting habit! Excessive strain on her thumbs had thrown her shoulders out of alignment, which shifted the position of her hips when she ran, which led to muscular strains elsewhere in her legs.

I'm not saying to become a monk who avoids all trappings of modern life and is always thinking about running. But long-term, you're going to better avoid the aches and pains of running if you're conscious of how you spend the bulk of your time affects your running body. All the things you've heard about good posture when sitting at a desk or driving, taking frequent breaks from the computer, having your work at eye level so that you're not straining to see or thrusting your head up or down and other matters of ergonomics become that much more important when you're a twenty-first century runner.

From the physician-heal-thyself department, I say this as someone with a tendency toward horrible posture. The better I am during the workday about sitting with good alignment and taking short breaks every hour, the better I feel on my post-work run.

112
Training Through Injury

Which injuries should you not run on, and which ones can you try to train through? The quick answer is that there's no quick answer. Because they're overuse injuries, almost all running injuries progress through degrees of severity. At the outset, they're mostly little pangs of discomfort. While you could play it safe and stop running until the pang disappears, you could wind up missing a lot of running that way. Plus, many of these little pangs are just white noise that go away 10 minutes into a run, never to be heard again. Most of the time, at least in the initial stages, keep running, while being ready to compromise on distance and pace at all times.

The one exception I'd make to this general guidance concerns stress fractures, which I'll discuss in more detail later in this chapter. You simply can't finesse your way through a stress fracture. One of your bones has a slight crack in it and needs to heal. At the best, running on it will delay that healing. In most cases, running on it will increase the size of the slight crack. At the worst, running on it can cause an outright fracture, the sort that's clearly visible on an x-ray. Take it from someone who once ran on a stress fracture for close to two years: You can't outsmart this injury. By the time I reached that last stage of grieving, acceptance, my shin bone was nearly broken in two. It then took me a year to return to daily running. The next time I knew I had a stress fracture, I immediately stopped running. Four weeks later, I was back on the road.

113
When to Run, When to Rest

So let's say you have a running-related pain that's not a stress fracture. How to proceed?

If you don't have pain while running, but after, or when you get up in the morning, it's OK to try running normal mileage at your normal pace. But keep good notes about the pain's frequency and severity. And be honest with yourself about whether it's not bothering you at all when you run.

If you can feel the ache when you're running, but it doesn't get worse during your run, you can try to carry on as per usual. When in doubt, stick close to home in case things get worse during the run and you need to shorten the run. (If it's noticeable mostly at the start of your run, then it's probably some tightness that you can get rid of with some flexibility work.)

If the pain gets worse as you run, something serious, or at least on the verge of being serious, is going on. Limit your run to less than the amount of time it takes for things to start deteriorating, and start crafting a rehab plan. You'll probably want to add some cross-training so that you don't feel guilty about running less and be tempted to keep running your normal mileage.

If the ache makes you alter your running form, you shouldn't be running on it. Doing so will not only delay healing of what's obviously a bad injury, but will also likely lead to injury elsewhere as your body compensates for your altered gait. In this case, it's time to find a cross-training activity that doesn't reproduce the running-related discomfort.

If the pain is present not only when you run but also during most of the day, you've let things go on for too long. You shouldn't run and should cross-train only if you can honestly say the activity produces no symptoms.

114

Dancing the Injury Limbo

Unless you're highly motivated or oblivious to pain or mule-headed (and yes, it can be hard to distinguish among those traits at times), most of your running injuries are going to be in those early stages, where how to proceed is based on judgment calls and guesstimation.

How much or whether to cut back in those cases will depend on lots of factors. Do you have an important race coming up in a month? In that case, you might be more inclined to stop for a day or two to see if that will calm what's become a persistent ache. That way, if the time off pretty much takes care of things, then you can get right back into race training. Of course, if you're in a non-race phase, then there's not as much urgency to preserving your fitness, so it could be easy to get yourself to take some downtime to let things heal.

Then again, you could make the argument (I certainly have!) that, with no important races in the near future, it's OK if this little limbo injury continues on for longer than it otherwise might if I stopped running on it. Especially if I'm going through a stressful period in other parts of my life, I'm willing to take a chance that a little strain won't get any worse by running on it so that I can get the stress relief that running brings. In that case I'm aware that I'm probably prolonging the time it will take to be free of the niggle, but it's worth it to me.

This sort of on-the-one-hand-on-the-other-hand discussion with yourself is, unfortunately, part of being a runner with any sort of injury. It's why being hurt is so mentally draining and is reason alone to do your best to avoid getting hurt in the first place.

115
The Doctor Will See You Now

But chances are he or she won't be all that helpful if you show up with a running injury. Most doctors aren't trained in sports medicine, and most aren't going to have insight into why you got injured, how to quickly overcome it, and how to avoid it in the future. I say this as someone who has running doctors for friends who would agree with all of the above.

At the minimum, see only doctors who have sports medicine certification in their fields. That will greatly increase your chances of them taking a holistic approach to solving your injury puzzle. And it should increase the chance that you'll get empathy on wanting to quickly return to action (instead of "If it hurts when you run, then don't run," or, "No wonder you're hurt—that's a lot of running!").

Word of mouth from other runners in your area is the best way to find a medical professional who can help. Podiatrists and osteopaths are often your best choices for finding a satisfying relationship as a runner. Chiropractors are trained to take a full-body view when looking for answers, but be wary if the answer involves repeated visits instead of a long-term do-at-home plan.

116

Pop Pills Prudently

If you have a new, acute running-related pain, it's OK to gobble ibuprofen or other anti-inflammatories in the first few days to see if that will get the inflammation under control. But if you're leaning on the pills to keep your running habit going, then it's time to step back and accept that you have an underlying injury issue that needs to be addressed. I have a friend who's been keeping the ibuprofen industry in business for the last fifteen years through his efforts to lessen chronic Achilles pain. And guess what? He still has the Achilles problem; if anything, it's gotten worse. (And who knows what's become of kidneys in this time.)

By the way, don't take anti-inflammatories just because you're a little sore after a long or hard run. The low-grade swelling that you sometimes feel after a killer session is part of your body's adaptation process. Leave it to resolve on its own, and you'll reap more of the benefits of that hard workout.

117

Ice Is Nice, Heat Can Be Hell

Consider ice your first line of defense against all running injuries. Ice any little niggle that doesn't go away during a run. In that case, five minutes of icing is plenty. If your niggle has deteriorated into something more like pain, then ice the area for five minutes after running, then again for five minutes an hour later. Also try to ice it one or two other times during the day. Icing will less the bad inflammation that accompanies a nascent injury, which is different than the good inflammation that can follow a hard but niggle-free session.

Don't heat a painful area after a run. Doing so will only increase swelling in the already inflamed soft tissues. Heat is best for areas that are tight, which is different than sore or inflamed. For tight areas, gentle heat (moist heat is best) can increase blood flow to soft tissue, which should increase range of motion in the area. Warm baths are fine (and fun) after something taxing like a long run if you wait long enough for any immediate post-run swelling to subside.

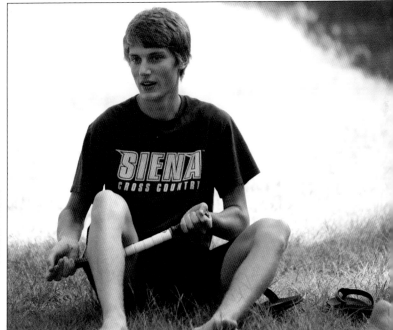

: Alison Wade

118

Massage, from Others and Yourself

Everybody agrees that massage feels great, but does it help prevent running injuries? Of course double-blind scientific studies are impossible to conduct on this matter. But there's plenty of evidence that a good deep-tissue massage can increase blood flow, which should help remove waste products from an injured area.

On the preventative side, I'll take the anecdotal observation that lots of elite runners get weekly massages as proof enough that it can help keep a running body healthy. If you can afford it, regular deep-tissue work can be part of your pre-hab program, where you do what you can to build your body's immunity to injury.

Self-massages like the Stick or foam rollers are great for getting some of these benefits on your own. Some areas (calves and quads) are easier to tend to than others. (After almost 20 years of using one, I've yet to figure out how to use the Stick on my lower back without increasing muscular tension elsewhere.) It's easy to overdo it with these things, so err on the side of caution—no more than 5 minutes on any one area. Apply pressure only to the point of a that's-the-stuff sensation; leave the hurts-so-good sensation for a trained therapist to produce. Stop immediately if applying pressure in one area causes you to feel sensations elsewhere.

119

Home Help: Plantar Fasciitis

While you're having tenderness in your heel and arch, baby the area. Keep a pair of slippers by the side of the bed that you can get into immediately. Several times a day, ice your heel and arch. The best choice is a frozen water bottle that you can roll the area over. This not only gets you the desired circular icing, but also works in a little massage. Before you run, loosen up the soft tissue along the bottom of your foot by grabbing the ball of your foot and pushing your toes toward your shin and back several times.

Long-term, plantar fasciitis is a sign that you should improve your calf and Achilles strength and flexibility. You'll probably also benefit from gradually moving away from running shoes that have a large drop from heel to forefoot.

120

Home Help: Achilles Tendinitis

Ice and anti-inflammatories are your short-term friends when your Achilles tendon is inflamed. The anti-inflammatories are especially helpful because blood flow to the tendon is limited, so it can be tough to get relief solely with icing. While you have Achilles tendinitis, put a slight heel lift in your non-running shoes to take some of the pressure off the tendon; corrugated cardboard, swapped a couple of times a day once it starts to compress, works well.

Same deal here as with plantar fasciitis: Getting Achilles tendinitis usually means you need to improve range of motion in the tendon and your calves. Part of that is not wearing heeled shoes during your non-running hours. In your running shoes, be sure the heel counter doesn't rub your Achilles tendon.

121

Home Help: Shin Splints

"Shin splints" is the lay term for medial tibial stress syndrome (which sounds even worse). Long-term, probably the best way to prevent shin splints is to keep running—it's mostly new runners or people returning to running after a long layoff who get them. If you do have frequent shin pain despite consistent running, then strengthen your arches (through walking barefoot around the house) so that your shin muscles don't have to pick up the slack for them when you run.

If you're having a bout of shin pain, run on soft surfaces if possible, and avoid downhills to lessen the pounding. Try to keep running, albeit less than usual if necessary, to keep the consistency that should eventually help you leave shin splints behind.

122

Home Help: Runner's Knee

While you're having pain around your kneecap, eliminate elements that require the knee to do extra stabilizing work. Run on flat, even surfaces, stay off of tracks and twisting trails, and avoid downhills. Runner's knee (patellofemoral pain syndrome to the medicos) is a good injury to finesse your way through on a treadmill. Putting the treadmill on a slight uphill grade should relieve some of the pressure on the knee.

Weak hips and glutes have been shown to be a key factor in developing running-related knee pain, because the knee tries to pick up some of the stabilizing work the muscles of your

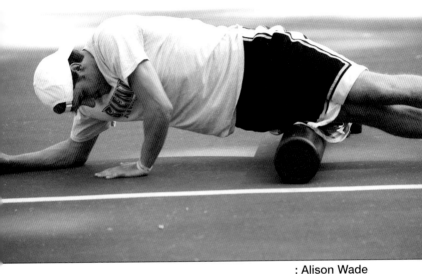

: Alison Wade

midsection are supposed to be doing. Every runner should devote time to building stronger hips, but especially those with one or more episodes of knee pain.

123
Home Help: Iliotibial Band Syndrome

Self massage, especially with a foam roller or device like the Stick, is really helpful here to loosen up the aggravated tendon. You'll also want to avoid the sorts of situations that may have brought on the pain in the first place—stay on level surfaces, or if you must run on slanted roads, switch sides often. If you're trying to finesse your way through this injury but still doing track workouts, then jog your recoveries going the opposite direction so that you're not always taking the turns with the same leg. (If you're blessed with an otherwise unoccupied track, alternate directions on your hard repeats.)

As with runner's knee, good hip and glute strength is important to preventing a recurrence. One-legged squats are good for strengthening your hip abductors, the ones on the outside of your hip that are supposed to stabilize you when your foot lands.

124
Home Help: Hamstring/Glute Pain

Tightness, tenderness and slight strains in the upper hamstrings and butt are going to be the bane of most ambitious runners at some point, especially ones who sit a lot in their non-running time. (Yes, that again! It really is significant.) During a flare-up, avoid steep uphills, and ease into all your runs. Make sure you're fully warmed up before hard workouts. If the sensation is of tenderness rather than tightness, don't stretch the area while it's in an acute phase, as that will just further irritate the already strained muscle fibers. Ice the area after all runs.

Once the acute tenderness is gone, be relentless about stretching your hip rotators and hamstrings, but never to the point that you reproduce the pain. Strengthening your hamstrings with single-leg curls will help to restore the proper balance of strength between your quads and hamstrings. And do what you can in your non-running time to sit with good posture and to get out of sitting postures at least once an hour.

125
Home Help: Stress Fractures

Again, you can't negotiate your way through a stress fracture. You have to stop running to let the bone heal. Sorry.

When you resume running, expect some discomfort, but not pain, where the fracture was. As long as the sensation there is more of a dull tug than a sharp pain, it's OK to gradually build back up. In some cases you might also have a bump where the fracture was; this is new bone that was laid down around the site of the fracture. I have one on my left shin. It's not the prettiest thing in the world, but it's not a source of pain (or concern). If anything, it's a visual reminder to never again get a stress fracture.

If you get more than one stress fracture, then you're repeatedly overloading one of your body's weak points. Lessen the chance of recurrence by being diligent about flexibility and strength work so that you're more resilient. Also, make sure your diet includes enough calcium.

126
Cross-training Caveat 1

When you're hurt and have to cross-train, try to spend more time on it than you do your running. After all, you can get in a decent run in 30 minutes, but you're not going to find lots of cyclists who would consider half an hour anything but a warm-up. Make the time go faster on individual workouts by translating your usual hard running workouts—VO$_2$ max sessions, tempo workouts, etc.—to the pool or bike or elliptical or wherever you're spending your non-running time. Structure crosstraining weeks like your running weeks; the variety will help your time in injury limbo pass faster than if you do the same medium-effort waiting-out-the-clock effort every day.

127
Do Something! Anything!

You'll probably spend the time you're hurt feeling like you're getting less fit and more fat by the hour. If your layoff from injury is long enough, you will indeed have a readjustment period once you resume running, no matter how dedicated you are with cross-training. So don't make things worse by an order of magnitude by wallowing in self-pity and apathy and not crosstraining. If you gain significant weight while you're on the shelf, the return to running will only be that much harder.

128
Cross-training Caveat 2

What's the best type of cross-training when you're injured? The first criteria is that it does not aggravate your injury. Doing the elliptical trainer if you have a stress fracture in your foot, for example, will just prolong your recovery.

After that, the most important criteria isn't which activity most closely mimics the mechanics of running or makes it easiest to keep your heart rate elevated. It's simpler than that: Which one are you most likely to do with the greatest regularity? Deep-water running, especially if you do hard intervals, is an excellent kissing-cousin substitute for real running. But if the closest pool is 20 miles away and allows deep-water running only at 6:00 AM, well, come on, let's be realistic about how often you'll get there. Of the obvious choices—deep-water running, cycling, using an elliptical trainer, using a stair machine—pick the ones that are most convenient for you to do daily.

129

It's Always a Good Time to Establish Good Habits

Among the positives to try to pull out of an injury bout: Treat it as a time when you improve your ancillary exercise routines—stretching, strengthening, core work, yoga, even meditation. It will feel good to know you're doing something to make your body more resistant to injury, and it should be relatively easy to stick with the routines once you're able to run again.

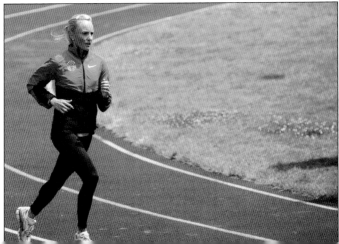

: Joel Wolpert

130

Running Form and Injury

In general people worry too much about running form as it relates to injury. By that I don't mean that running form doesn't matter. It does—a lot. But bad running form is more an indicator that you have something going on that can lead to injury than a primary cause of injury.

That is, let's say when you run your feet splay out to the side. (Check this the next time you run through snow or with wet shoes on dry pavement.) That flaw in your form will certainly make you slower and could lead to other form issues as your body attempts to compensate. But the original matter of splayed feet is a secondary matter stemming from tightness or weakness in your body. (In this case, most likely tight hip flexors, the muscles along the front top of your thighs.) That weakness is leading to the bad aspect of running form, and that weakness might very well over time cause compensations elsewhere in your body that will lead to injury, often not where the original problem is.

So the way to think about good running form as it relates to injury isn't to obsess over how you're running all the time and monitoring yourself with every step. Rather, as you notice deviations from the basics of good running form, take those as signs of weakness or tightness that need to be addressed. When you successfully improve those underlying weaknesses or tightnesses, the form issues should go away on their own without you having to be constantly conscious of them.

131

What's Good Running Form?

There's no one universally desirable running form, any more than you would expect all baseball players to have the same swing. We each run the way we do because of the unique way our bodies are put together—the length of our torso in relation to our legs, the shape of our feet, the alignment of our bones, the communication between our brain and central nervous system, and a million other things.

So you run the way you do for some inherent reasons, and to a certain extent, you shouldn't try to change that. At the same time, we all have a range of how well our unique form manifests itself. When you have weakness or tightness in one or more places in your body, your unique form will move toward the less desirable end of its range. Probably when you were a kid, especially if you had an active childhood, your form was toward the more desirable end of its range.

By building a stronger, more supple running body, you can ensure that you'll usually be moving with the more desirable version of your running form. That's going to include your personal version of these elements of good form: landing over your center of gravity; a light, rapid cadence; minimal lateral rotation; and easier to spot than quantify, relaxed body position.

132
Form Flaw: Tight Shoulders and Neck

When your shoulders and neck are tight, you tend to run with your shoulders hunched and your arms held out to the side. You probably also look like you have a short neck. Running like this keeps your arms from flowing back and forth, which affects your leg turnover, and simply wastes energy on holding your arms in an unnatural manner.

Perhaps you won't be surprised by now to hear this is a form flaw we can pin on modern life. Hour upon hour in front of a computer or other screen tends to cause you to sit with your shoulders tight and hunched. Those postural habits tend to carry over to when it's time to run. Good posture and ergonomics can help eliminate that chronic tightness, and simple mindfulness while you're running can help relax your shoulders and neck until you get them to be so normally. Concentrate on having your wrists pass by your waist.

133
Form Flaw: Head Thrust Forward

You want your head directly over your body, not out in front like a search party. When you run with your head thrust forward, your neck and upper back muscles have to tighten to maintain the head's position, a waste of energy that has nothing to do with moving down the road quickly and efficiently.

This form flaw is yet another curse of modernity, brought on by straining our heads forward to look at some screen or another that's too far away. (Or that would be the right distance away if we would admit our eyesight isn't what it used to be.) Again, get the ergonomics of your computer set up right. In the meantime, before runs lie on your back and tuck your chin to your chest ten times to reset your head position. While running, try to stay conscious of your head floating weightlessly over your shoulders.

134
Form Flaw: Excessive Forward Lean

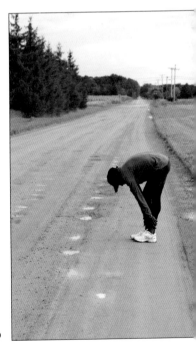

Running bent over from the waist means that your lower back has to work to hold you up, and your quads have to work extra to keep you from falling forward. So you run less efficiently, you tire more easily, and your legs can become unnecessarily sore.

Too much sitting is usually the culprit here, gradually robbing your lower back of the small curve it used to have. (Look at race photos and you'll see that almost every runner who leans forward from the waist is in the older age groups.) In addition to sitting so that your lower back is arched, you can fight this problem by strengthening your abs and butt.

: Stacey Cramp

135

Form Flaw: Excessive Lateral Rotation

When your trunk is unstable, your arms and legs start moving in directions other than straight ahead. With every step, you're using energy to bring your arms and legs back toward the midline of your body instead of moving them forward. This problem is usually caused by weak abs and butt muscles. Strengthen those key postural stabilizers, and more of your motion will be directed in front of you rather than to the side. Put another way, for the same energy cost, you'll run faster.

136

Form Flaw: Splayed Feet

To some degree, how much of a straight line your feet land and push off in is genetic; if you were born with less-than-ideal bone alignment in your legs, then your feet will probably splay some. But there's undoubtedly a fixable element here as well. If your butt muscles are weak and/or your hip flexors are tight (the two often go together), then your foot placement while running will probably be compromised. Splayed feet is a great example of a problem you'll more successfully improve long-term by fixing your underlying running structure than by consciously trying to better while running. (Trust me, as someone whose right foot points out when he gets tired, I can tell you it doesn't work to try to force it to land straight.)

137
Essential Extras

Think of the items I'm about to discuss—flexibility and strengthening—not in either/or terms in relation to your running, but in terms of "yes, and ... " That is, they're not replacements for running, but a form of insurance policy that will allow you to better pursue and enjoy your running at whatever level you choose to. Even if they don't improve your performance—and they almost certainly will—when done correctly they're going to make the simple act of running feel better, especially the older you get and the longer you've been running. Most of these activities are easy to sneak in throughout the day in little clumps of activity.

138
Why to Stretch

All runners benefit from good range of motion throughout the body so that running is a smooth, flowing activity. When it's not, not only do you run slower, but the compromised motion eventually leads to compensation elsewhere in the body, setting off a bad kinetic chain that will lead to further deterioration and, usually, injury. For almost all modern runners, extra work will be necessary to retain the desired degree of flexibility, and that's almost always going to mean doing regular stretching.

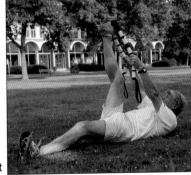

: 101° West

139
How to Stretch

B ut what kind? static? ballistic? dynamic?
Based on research and what top runners do, and years of experimentation on my own, I'm convinced that the best type of stretching for runners is a technique known as active isolated stretching (AIS). The technique is based on the premise that muscles work in opposing pairs (quads and hamstrings, biceps and triceps, and so on). To most effectively stretch one of the muscles in the pair, the theory goes, contract its opposite. So to stretch your hamstrings, contract your quad while raising your straight leg from the ground. This allows the hamstrings to relax and gradually lengthen, in contrast to being forced through a range of motion that can cause them to reflexively protect against over-stretching by constricting.

AIS combines elements of static and dynamic stretching. For each muscle you're stretching, you do 10 or so stretches, pausing only at the very end of the stretch, with each stretch lasting only a few seconds. For most of the stretches, you use a rope to assist at the end of the stretch for just a little bit more range of motion.

Among runners, AIS has been popularized by the father-and-son team of Jim and Phil Wharton. I highly recommend their books and videos, as do some of the best distance runners of the last fifteen years.

SCOTT DOUGLAS

140

Other Types of Flexibility Work

That's not to say AIS is the only type of stretching (just probably the most effective at permanently increasing range of
motion). The old standby of static stretching is certainly better
than nothing. Research has pretty conclusively shown that, for
runners, it's best saved for after running. Holding stretches for the
prescribed 30 seconds before a run can cause a decrease in the
stretched muscle's power in the near future, which is hardly what
you want before a hard workout.

Before a run, the best non-AIS stretches are dynamic movements that prepare your body for the range of motion it will move
through out on the roads. Activities like leg swings and walking
with high knees will help you start your runs readier to move efficiently. The key is to ease into each one so that your muscles don't
constrict protectively from suddenly being thrust into action.

141

What About Yoga?

Because of the sustained poses, yoga isn't ideal soon before
running. (See above about lessened muscle power following
static stretching.) But I'm certainly not going to discourage any
runner from an activity that can increase flexibility, balance, and
body awareness.

Probably the greatest benefit of yoga for runners comes from
balance poses, like the Tree. These help strengthen the small stabilizing muscles in your hips and butt that play a large role in

117

running economically. The biggest caveat for a runner going into a yoga session is to always be mindful that you're a runner first. In a class, you're likely to be around people with greater flexibility on many poses, and the idea isn't to will your body into positions it can't currently handle to show off how fit you are. Go only to the point of gentle opening, regardless of what others around you or on the video you're following along with are doing.

142

When to Stretch: Part 1

The gold standard is a complete stretching routine before and after every run. Now let's deal in reality.

Before most runs, spend at least a few minutes on the muscles on the back of your body—calves, hamstrings, glutes, lower back. They're the muscles that are going to be shortest and tightest from the last several hours of your life. Active isolated stretching or dynamic stretching is the way to go pre-run. If you've been sitting for the last while before your run, do the Cat-Cow exercise: On your hands and knees, round your back and draw your belly button toward the ceiling while tucking your chin (cat), then arch your back and raise your gaze to the ceiling (cow). Doing a cycle of this exercise will loosen the soft tissue around your pelvis and allow you to start your run feeling more fluid.

After running, spend a few minutes on any areas that felt tight or otherwise troublesome on the run. Hips, glutes, and hamstrings appreciate a little attention at this point. Active isolated stretching is good at this time; if you're a fan of static stretching, post-run is the time for it. If you drove to run, when you get out of the car, do Cat-Cow to help unlock your pelvis.

143

When to Stretch: Part 2

Little bouts of stretching pre- and post-run will help you on individual runs, but they're more about maintaining flexibility than improving it. For the latter, you need a few longer sessions of 15–20 minutes each, a few times a week. If you can do these in the two hours before a run, great.

Otherwise, find a few blocks during the week for this essential insurance payment. If you don't run every day, then your non-running days are an obvious opportunity. Another easily claimed block is a weekend afternoon, especially if you've run long in the morning. Early in the morning on a workday, or midday if you can find a suitable location, are also times when others might leave you along long enough for you to get something good done for yourself. Finally, a brief session soon before going to bed when the rest of your responsibilities for the day are taken care of is a nice way to unwind and end the day.

And bear in mind that you can sneak in little bouts of stretching throughout your day. You can do foot circles (described below) sitting at your desk. You can take a short break and instead of listen to someone blab about what they watched on TV last night, loosen your shoulders and neck (also described below). Continually stretching during these "stolen" times will help keep you loose enough that more dramatic intervention, in the form of several long stretching sessions each week, won't be as necessary.

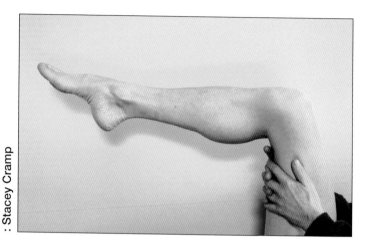

: Stacey Cramp

144

The Obvious Stuff to Stretch

Most runners intuitively know to work on the large muscle groups involved in running—calves, hamstrings, hips, quads, glutes. If your calves are fairly tight, stretch them first, because once they're loosened up, you can better target your hamstrings.

145

Feet and Ankle Flexibility

Good range of motion in your feet and ankles would seem to be a no-brainer, but a lot of runners ignore these areas.

Restricted flexibility in these joints can have a major negative cascade effect throughout your gait and will also make you slower.

Maintain strong, vibrant levers for your running stride with regular foot and ankle work. Gas pedals, in which you flex your foot down and up as if flooring a car accelerator, and foot circles, in which you rotate your foot clockwise, then counterclockwise several times, are great. They're the sort of stretch that's easy to sneak in a few times a day while you're otherwise in non-running mode. Sitting at home, perhaps while reading or watching TV, you can tend to the balls of your feet: Grab your toes and move them up and down.

146
Upper-Body Flexibility

Many of the form flaws we looked at earlier stem from a tight upper body. Increase your chances of running with a smooth whole-body motion by maintaining good upper-body flexibility. The shoulders are key here—think of them as your arms' hips in which you want good range of motion in all directions. Do stretches that target the different shoulder muscles, such as internal and external rotators.

Also work on your neck so that you can hold your head loosely over your body when you run. Jim and Phil Wharton's materials show an excellent series of stretches for neck and shoulder muscles. As with the feet and ankle stretches, these are easy to sneak in a few times a day as a great way to reboot your body and counteract too much sitting, typing, and time in front of screens.

147

A Stronger Runner

Everybody should do some form of strength training, just like everybody should do some form of cardiovascular exercise. What I'm going to focus on here is the type of strength training that's most relevant for building an injury-resistant running body. And that means targeted exercises that are often different than what you would do if your strength training goal was to see how much you could bench-press or look good at the beach. Spend your limited time focusing on the muscles that most often get weak and tight from the repetitive nature of running combined with, that's right, the insults to the running body that modern life induces.

148

Leg Strengthening

The most important areas to target are your knee extensors, hip adductors, hip abductors, hip flexors, hip extensors, gluteals, soleus, and gastrocnemius.

Three sets of 10 reps with light weights is the prescription here. The emphasis is on isolating the targeted muscle so you don't want to heave around as much weight as possible, because that would encourage supporting muscles to kick in and do some of the work. Remember, the goal is to strengthen specific, often minor muscles, not to build your overall strength and general buffitude.

For example, let's say I'm targeting my knee extensors (thigh muscles above the knee toward the midline of the body). I do these seated, with an 8-pound ankle weight, straightening my lower leg by contracting my knee extensors. The sensation in the muscles I'm targeting is of a little extra work than if I were extending my leg without the weights. Of course I could do the same exercise with more than three times the weight, but at some point, to raise my leg I'd start recruiting hip muscles and other quad muscles than the ones I'm targeting.

Aim for two to three leg strengthening sessions per week, ideally on your easiest running days.

149
Upper-Body Strengthening

Most of the relevant upper-body muscles are along the back of your body. Sorry, but these mostly aren't the ooh-and-ah aren't-I-ripped flex muscles. The most important areas to target are your deltoids, pectoralis majors, triceps, shoulder external rotators, shoulder internal rotators, trapezius, and rhomboids. These muscles help you to maintain an upright, relaxed posture while running, giving you a smoother, more flowing stride.

Same deal as with legs on reps, sets, and what might seem like too-low weights. Aim for two to three sessions per week. The weights are light enough that they shouldn't interfere with the quality of your runs, so do the work whenever you can find the time.

150
Midsection Strengthening

Much of what people consider core training is covered by the leg strengthening exercises I listed above. Those hip and butt exercises will give you great stability in your pelvic area, resulting in less impact stress on other parts of your body.

For your midsection, there are a million theories on how best to proceed. For busy runners looking to spend their time efficiently on exercises with relevance to their sport, you could do worse than getting in the habit of doing a series of plank poses after running. Thirty seconds to a minute for each of prone plank, supine plank, and right and left side plank is a good goal. Do that most days and over time you'll be better off than people who have overly ambitious, overly complex routines that they stop doing sooner or later. (Usually sooner.)

If you want to be more ambitious about a midsection strengthening routine, the elite coaches Greg McMillan and Jay Johnson have each produced excellent DVDs showing which of the infinite potential exercises have the greatest relevance for runners.

151
General Strength Exercises

An increasing number of top runners do regular routines of what they call "general strength" exercises. By that they mean Pilates-meets-football-practice exercises like leg lifts, one-leg squats, push-ups with a clap, lunges, etc. The theory is that modern life deprives children of the all-around general body fitness that agrarian lifestyles and unstructured play helped build fifty years ago. Without that type of fitness, the theory goes, you're much more susceptible to injury once you devote yourself to the one-directional movement patterns of running. General strength exercises build that fitness that used to be taken for granted.

You probably won't be surprised to hear I think the theory makes sense, especially for adult runners who are sedentary all day except when they run. For many people, the issue will come down to time: Can you find time to run and stretch and do running-specific strengthening, and then find more time for general strength routines? If so, Jay Johnson is again your guide, and this time the resources are free: Go to runningtimes.com/gsvideos and you'll find five videos by Johnson detailing a progression of general strength routines.

152
Running Shoes and Injury

For years the running shoe industry has cast its products more or less like well, a cast: Wear this protective device or you're at serious risk of injury. Fortunately, that mind-set is starting to change; shoe companies and runners increasingly recognize that the goal of running shoes should be to allow the feet and ankles to do their thing with as little interference as possible. You hear a lot less these days than even five years ago about a shoe's "protective" qualities and more about how it enhances the body's natural mechanics.

That was a needed change—as if one of humanity's most basic movements was possible to do free from injury only if done in something mass-produced with foam and plastic in an Asian factory. If anything, many runners, including me, have considered most modern running shoes potential vectors of injury.

153

Minimalism: Is Less More?

For the most part, it's a good idea to do at least some of your running in light, flexible shoes.

What's been termed "minimalism" over the past few years is really what most runners naturally did before the shoe industry started pumping shoes full of technology, dramatically elevating the height of the midsole, and creating large differences between the midsole height in the heel and forefoot. Before shoes started resembling moon boots, most runners trained in low-to-the-ground models that hugged the foot. Combine that with doing hard workouts in racing flats, and you were doing most of your mileage in fairly minimal shoes. The benefits include stronger and more flexible feet and ankles; more, not less, stability (because you're closer to the ground rather than feeling suspended above it); encouragement of a lighter, quicker turnover; and simply enjoying running more because of a greater feel of the surface you're moving over.

154

Modern Minimalism

Now you have to make more of a conscious effort to get in shoes that don't feel like pillows on your feet. I'm not alone among longtime runners in doing much of my running in what are marketed as racing shoes, because what's now sold as a racing shoe is quite similar to what were sold as a lightweight training shoe twenty years ago.

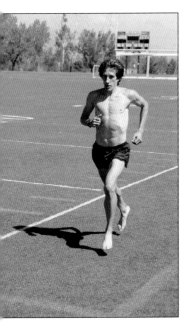

If you've always run in modern, overly built running shoes, experiment with running in less shoe. Get a pair of lightweight trainers and gradually mix them into your shoe rotation. Start doing striders and hard workouts in racing shoes. At first you might experience some calf and Achilles tightness as these body parts relearn how to do what they're supposed to do. But over time, if you're like most runners who have gone this route, you'll not want to return to the heavily cushioned shoes that too often get in the way of your run instead of getting out of the way and just letting you run.

155
Barefoot in the Park

If slight shoes are good, what about none? You might think from media reports that barefoot running was invented circa summer of 2009 and that it's some controversial practice that shoe companies want to remain hidden from runners. And for sure, in classic American fashion, proponents of barefoot running have taken the kernel of a solid idea and run with it past its logical extreme.

The truth is, barefoot running has been part of many runners' training for decades, even among those sponsored by shoe companies. Coaches have long recommended barefoot striders on the infield of a track or a grass field to build foot and ankle strength and flexibility. It's quite possible (and enjoyable) to quickly, safely build to doing 30 minutes or more of barefoot running on forgiving surfaces. (In high school, I did a barefoot 14-miler via repeated loops of my school's grass perimeter. It's still one of the most enjoyable solo runs in my three-decade running career.) Most runners for at least a few warm months a year can find somewhere sensible to regularly incorporate a couple barefoot sessions a week into their training.

As in almost all areas of running, the thing to avoid is zealotry. In terms of barefoot running, that means avoiding doing too much too soon, especially if you've spent most of your life in overly built-up shoes, and not being an idiot about what surfaces you run barefoot on. At some point, the risks of sharp objects and hard asphalt outweigh the benefits of greater foot function if you start running most of your miles barefoot on the roads.

Going barefoot or in socks indoors as much as possible is an excellent way to get some of the benefits of barefoot running.

156
Tossing Your Trainers

When to replace your shoes is a judgment call that you'll get a better sense of the longer you run. The usual recommendation to replace shoes every 300 to 500 miles is based more on manufacturers' desires to move product than anything else. Thirty years ago, we were told to replace shoes every 500 miles. Every year since then, manufacturers have said how the latest shoes are new and improved, quite possibly the greatest shoes ever made. And yet they don't last longer than when Ronald Reagan was president? Come on.

The less built-up a shoe you run in, the less reason there is to discard them after a given number of miles, because there's that much less midsole cushioning to break down.

If you find you're unaccountably sore after several consecutive runs in the same shoes, that's a good sign that their retirement might be imminent. Certainly if they're so broken down that they're altering your gait, it's time to ditch them. This is usually from the heel counters being worn over to one side—if you place them on a level surface and you can get them to rock back and forth by flicking the midsole near the back, then it's probably time to move on.

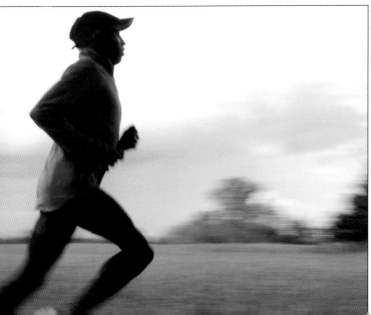

: Stacey Cramp

157

Orthotics Aren't a Cure-All

Don't look to orthotics as a permanent solution to injury, any more than you would look to crutches as a necessary companion for the rest of your life. If you've had orthotics for a long time, ask yourself: Do I still have the problem I originally got these for? Have I been diligent about improving my strength and flexibility so that the original problem doesn't recur?

If you decide to wean yourself off orthotics, start by gradually going without them during your non-running time. As you feel safe doing that, do one short run per week without them, then two and keep progressing as your body finds things agreeable.

158

Final Thought on Running Injuries

Do yourself a favor and stay at a good running weight. Given that with every running step you're landing with 3 to 4 times your bodyweight, unnecessary pounds put unnecessary strain on joints, ligaments, and bones.

PART FOUR

Running Consistently: 43 Tips to Help You Run More Often for the Rest of Your Life

It's not uncommon to go to bed thinking, "Darn, I should have run today." It's not common to go to bed thinking, "I shouldn't have run today."

Consistency is the runner's holy grail. Any good coach will tell you the biggest factor in running success is consistency. Without it, you're never going to come close to reaching your potential, either within a season, a year, or a decade. Or a lifetime, for that matter. You might have brief displays of brilliance, but until you learn how to pull off regular running that builds from day to day, week to week, month to month, year to year, you're not going to get very far.

After all, running isn't like, say, golf, where you can set it aside for two months and almost immediately be as good as you were your last time on the links. Running is more how the concert pianist Vladimir Horowitz described his relationship with music: "If I don't practice for a day," he said, "I know it. If I don't practice for two days, my wife knows it. If I don't practice for three days, the world knows it."

Don't worry, I'm not saying to run every day no matter what or don't bother. I'm saying that good running over the long-term has a rhythm, just like a good individual run does. Consistently running five days a week for two months is better than a month of running every day followed by a month of running twice a week. Running regularly at a level you can sustain throughout the seasons is better than training hard all fall and then bagging it during the winter. And running year to year with a steady-as-she-goes mind-set is better than two years of zealotry followed by retirement.

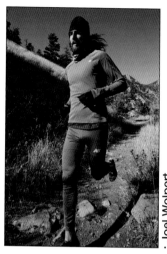

: Joel Wolpert

The tips in this chapter will help you achieve consistency throughout your running career, starting with the simple matter of what's often the biggest challenge: How to get yourself out the door today, and then again tomorrow. We'll also look at other challenges you'll likely face to achieving, for lack of a better term, consistent consistency: lack of motivation, weather, aging, and travel.

159

Number One Foe of Runners: Inertia

Mark Twain said that the secret to successful writing was to apply the seat of one's pants to the seat of a chair. The running corollary is to apply the bottom of your running shoes to the space just outside your front door. It really is that simple.

"Simple," of course, doesn't mean "easy." Inertia is one of the most powerful forces in the universe, or at least the part about a body at rest tending to stay at rest is. (I've often thought that Sir Isaac Newton should have tried a few more 20-milers before definitively stating that a body in motion stays in motion unless acted on by an external force.) The desire to go run, to do something so drastically different from how most of us spend our days, is highly appealing in the abstract, but can be difficult to conjure when you're already tired, or it's cold and dark outside, or twenty seven people are making what they say are critical demands on your time right now. In that moment, it's easy to justify avoiding the simple step of putting on your running shoes and stepping outside.

The best thing you can do about inertia, both on any given day and in a lifetime of running, is to acknowledge its power and then move on. Picture yourself going to bed that evening and reviewing the day. Will you be glad you ran? Yes, you almost certainly will. So defeat inertia and make that happen.

160

Finding Time

Thanks to my profession, appearance and frequent appearances in not much clothing on local roads, people tend to know I'm a runner. There's a subset of non-runners who (mistakenly) think I want to evangelize about running, and they try to preemptively stop that by saying something like, "I would like to run, but I don't have the time." And then they probably go home

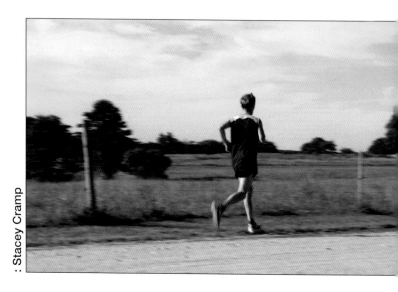

: Stacey Cramp

and watch TV for four hours or read updates from all 313 of their Facebook friends.

Because you're reading this book, I'm going to assume you know the "I don't have time" line is almost never true. You've experienced another of my idiot-savant-as-running-coach truisms: We find the time for the things that are important to us. Period.

161
Not If, but When

Put perhaps a little less harshly, what I mean is that if running is important to you (and I kinda think it should be), then your mind-set shifts from "Can I find the time for it?" to "When can I find the time for it?" You think in terms not of "Will I run today?" but "When will I run today?"

Because let's face it, whether you run today matters to almost nobody else in the world but you. Your boss, the dog, traffic, errands, your kids, your friends, a little extra sleep—the list of claims on your time is endless. To wait to see if an opening magically arrives in your day when you'll be able to run is to surrender your running to those claims on your time. And remember, almost none of those claims are going to care if you go to bed kicking yourself for missing a day of running. That's not to say they're evil or out to get you; they may very well love you. But they're still almost always going to request that you do something other than change into your running gear and disappear for the next little while.

So if there are lots of claims on your time, anticipate when you'll be able to run, and make it happen. During the work week, that will often mean getting a little less sleep and running early in the morning. So be it.

162

Running Ain't Needlework

One challenge to finding time to run is the nature of running—you need a solid block of time. Running regularly doesn't work like doing needlework or reading or even some physical pursuits, like ab exercises. You can't squeeze in a few minutes here, a few minutes there, and at the end of the day have made good progress.

Complicating matters is eating. Wouldn't it be fabulous, I've long thought, if running worked something like gardening, where

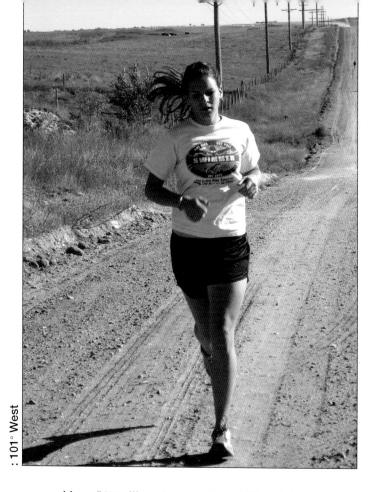

you could say, "OK, I'll eat dinner with the kids and then immediately after spend half an hour on my passion."

The need to find a solid block of time that doesn't conflict with yours and others' eating schedules is, I think, among the reasons running isn't more popular. But that just makes it that much more special for us, doesn't it?

163

If, on the Other Hand, You Have All Day

On what are probably the rare occasions when you could run at pretty much any time of the day, don't wait until you feel "ready" to run. You're almost never going to feel ready to run. I say this from too much experience during my idle youth—the stars are never going to align such that you're suddenly full of energy and a world-beating attitude. Lying on the couch for another hour isn't going to imbue you with eagerness; if anything, it will just make you more lethargic, and the day will have 60 minutes less in it. Just get out there and get on with your run.

164

Something Is Always Better Than Nothing

One impediment to success in consistency is taking an all-or-nothing approach to your running. You're asking for trouble, or at least disappointment, if you convince yourself that running has to happen in a certain way or otherwise not be worth it or legitimate.

There will be days when some aspect of reality intrudes and you have to scrap your ideal-world training plan. It could be weather or work or a family matter or fatigue or maybe just sleeping through your alarm. That doesn't make the logical conclusion to be scrapping the whole affair. A 4-miler is much closer to a 10-miler than it is to 0 miles for the day.

This is also an important idea to keep in mind once you're out running. Things aren't always going to go like they "should" or how you want them to. You might feel like you're hauling but be running much slower than usual. You might have a new niggle. Maybe the track you were going to do a workout on is locked. Don't draw dramatic conclusions or make dramatic decisions from single events. See the run through and hope for a better run tomorrow.

165

I ⊙ Running

A related habit of mind is to view your running like you do a committed relationship. You're in the relationship because you want to be and your life is better because of it. Yes, sometimes you're going to feel like you're doing all the work and getting

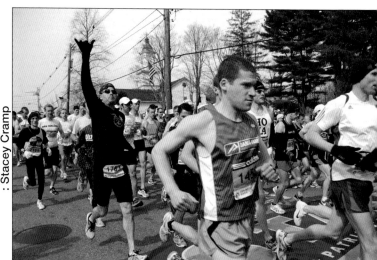

: Stacey Cramp

nothing in return. Little things might really irritate you. Others' relationships, or former relationships of yours, might look great from a distance. But that doesn't mean you just walk away from the relationship because you've hit a rough patch. Stay committed, and soon enough your devotion will be rewarded and you'll appreciate anew all that keeps you in the relationship.

166

Gotta Get a Goal

Marathon legend Bill Rodgers is a master at self-motivation. The thing that's kept him running ambitiously for the last four decades is that he's always working toward a goal. For Rodgers, that usually means a key race or series of races over the next three to six months. That's a short enough amount of time that the goal isn't so distant as to be abstract, but long-term enough that it provides impetus to his running in the weeks and months before, as it gives him something to look forward to achieving.

Rodgers' goals are always models of what sport psychologists say are good goals: personally meaningful, measurable, specific, challenging but within reach and tiered (meaning that it's easy to create short-term goals that build to the long-term goal). Eliminate any of those elements, and the goal doesn't serve as successful of a motivator. For example, remove the specificity aspect, and "I want to break 40:00 for 10K" becomes "I want to run faster for 10K." In the latter case, it's quite likely you could achieve your goal almost immediately, and then what?

One great thing about goals the way Rodgers sets them is that they give immediate meaning to what he runs daily. Knowing that he aims to run a certain time for a certain distance on a certain date, he then works backward from that date and creates a training plan that builds logically to achieving that goal. What he does today is informed by where he is on the path to that goal as well as what he did last week and what he'll do next week to meet it.

167
It Doesn't Have to Be a Race Goal

Of course, there are excellent running goals that have nothing to do with race performance but that meet all the criteria for ones that will provide impetus and inspiration.

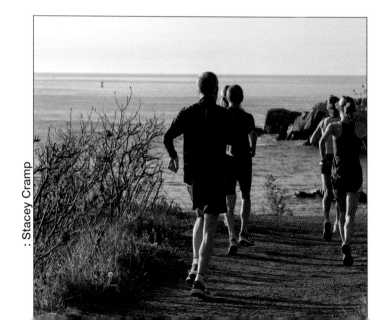

: Stacey Cramp

For example, every year on January 1, when I write my goals for the year, the first one is "Miss no days to injury." That's not just an aspiration. It's a quantifiable goal that motivates me to do regular body-maintenance work (stretching, strengthening, core work, etc.) so that I'm more resistant to injury. It also helps me to remain mindful of not making stupid training errors, like four hard days in a row, so that I'm not looking back ten days later shaking my head in disgust at the hamstring strain that seemingly came out of nowhere. You might find equal motivation from a goal like "Average 40 miles a week for the year" or "Run at least five days a week for the next three months."

If you can always state with specificity what your current running goal is, and if that goal is something you picked because it has real meaning to you, then you've gone a long way to ensuring consistency in your running.

168
The Greatest Running Invention Ever

Here's another insight from the master of running psychology, Bill Rodgers: The single best thing you can do to ensure consistency in running is to get yourself one or more good training partners.

Training partners will make it infinitely easier to achieve all of the habits of success I've described above. They'll get you out the door. They'll make your time for running seem more legitimate to yourself and others because it will be viewed as an appointment. They'll keep you out there when the going gets tough. They'll be sounding boards for and aids to formulating and progressing toward your goals.

It's impossible to say enough good things about good training partners. The runners who have reached their potential completely on their own are by far the exceptions.

Performance aside, nurturing a pool of training partners will help your running simply because it will help your life. A few hours together a week on the road will forge friendships of a quality that are hard to initiate elsewhere in normal adult life.

169
Dancing with Your Partner(s)

Not all of your training partners need to be of your speed and typical mileage. People of roughly your ilk are your bread-and-butter partners, but there's no reason to avoid runners who are significantly faster or slower, or who run a lot less or more than you do.

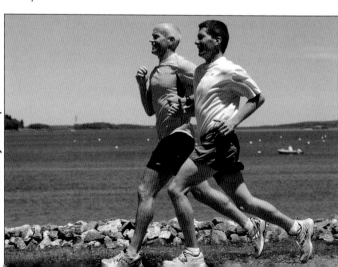

: Stacey Cramp

If someone is much slower than you, plan to run with him on the day after your hardest workout of the week. If someone is much faster than you, then latch on to her normal run and use it as a tempo run. If someone is going half as far as you usually go, do his run and then add on. If someone is a mileage maniac, join her for the first part of her run. All these runners will welcome your company.

170
Running Partners of a Different Sort

Become a student of the sport. Read biographies of great runners. Find a running message board that features knowledgeable (and ideally, nonabusive) runners. Why, you could even subscribe to the magazine I work for! It ruins none of the magic of self-discovery to learn that thousands of others have gone before you and experienced every challenge and joy that you have. Take advantage of the lessons others have drawn from their mistakes so that you don't have to repeat them.

171
Sick and Tired (But Not of Running)

At some point, getting sick is going to get in the way of your running. The usual advice is that it's OK to keep running if your symptoms are from the neck up (runny nose, woozy head, etc.), but that you shouldn't run if your symptoms are below your head (congestion in chest, coughing, vomiting, etc.).

Like so much in running, however, running when you're sick is a judgment call, not a black-and-white matter. I almost always at least attempt a token jog, on the theory that half an hour after the run I might feel significantly better than I did before. The run is unlikely to be a peak experience, but it's something different than sitting around with a box of tissues, and I usually feel a little cleared out from the increased blood flow. I stay close to home in case it becomes obvious 10 minutes into the run that further escapades are contraindicated. But even on those occasions, it's hard to argue that a short jog was a mistake—it's not like doing so will have made you that much sicker or delayed your recovery.

Again, this is a judgment call. Some of us just like to run pretty much every day. I like the thought that the cold or flu, which is already lowering my quality of life, didn't completely upend things.

172
Diet and Regularity

By which I mean running regularity, not the type usually associated with diet.

The most important reason to care about your diet as a runner isn't so you can run 8 seconds faster in a 5K or run 21 miles instead of 19 next Sunday. It's so that you have basic underlying good health to use as a platform for regular running. It's tough to maintain good running habits if you're always getting sick or overly fatigued or feeling like you're always on the verge of coming down with something. By helping to impart a basic level of good health, a good diet will allow you to run more consistently and ambitiously.

That being the case, what constitutes a good running diet is pretty much what constitutes a good diet, period: Lots of fresh fruits and vegetables; small servings of lean protein; plenty of high-quality carbs to keep your muscles fueled; plenty of fluids not pumped full of sugar; easy on the saturated fat and processed foods. It really is that simple, despite the machinations and manipulations and faddish focuses you'll hear encouraged.

If you want to take a basic daily multivitamin as a form of insurance for occasional poor dietary choices, fine. Other supplements advertised as being beneficial to runners are a waste of your money.

People like to say, "I'm a runner, so I can eat whatever I want." And that can be true, if your only concern about your diet is a simple calories-in/calories-out calculation. Me, I would prefer to feel as well as possible throughout the day and when running. That's going to happen with a lot more regularity if those calories mostly come from simple, healthful foods whose ingredients I know how to pronounce without a degree in chemistry.

173
Weather the Weather

Running consistently also means running through all kinds of weather. (Unless you live somewhere like, say, San Diego, where you have to adapt to it being sunny and 72 when just the other day it was sunny and 78.) Succeeding in running throughout all the seasons is mostly a matter of your mental outlook, with the right clothing choices in a supporting role.

Through lack of exposure and a Weather Channel ethos that portrays climate as something that descends from above to prey on us, most people are weather wimps. Run long enough, and you'll eventually be asked after some non–San Diego day, "Really? You run in this?" What these people don't realize is that one of the great joys of being a runner is experiencing nature through all the seasons. The variety of temperature and how the air feels and quality of light, whether trees are in bloom or the leaves are starting to fall, those sorts of things make running outside year-round a treat that most people don't appreciate until they experience it.

When given reason to be, humans are amazingly adaptive to a wide range of climates. So, yes, I do "run in this." So should you. The weather is never as bad as it appears from the other side of your office or car window.

174

Weather Wimpiness

A simple test: On days when you're struggling to get out the door, ask yourself, "Would I be thinking like this if it were 75 and sunny?" If the answer is no, then that's seldom a sufficient reason to skip a run. (In other words, runners in San Diego never to get to miss a day because of the weather.) Of course this doesn't mean you're not allowed to complain about the weather. Do like I do—get your bitching in, and then get going.

175

Running Hot

There's a reason places like Louisiana and Saudi Arabia aren't distance-running hotbeds, so to speak. Distance-running performance starts to decline when you've lost as little as 2 percent of your bodyweight to dehydration. That's sweating away only 3 pounds for a 150-pound runner, which can easily happen in less than an hour's run. Those of us who are heavy sweaters can lose much more, setting off a downward spiral of shallow breathing, soaring heart rate, and dramatic slowing. Take it from someone who once went from 130 to 121 pounds during a two-hour July run: Despite the long hours of daylight and the joy of not having to bundle up to brave the elements, maintaining high-quality running can be toughest in the summer.

For overall consistency, the challenge isn't so much getting out the door on any given day. It's summer, after all, and it's almost always pleasant to step outside. The challenge is more keeping on top of how drained running in the heat can leave you so that you do more than muddle through until the first crisp fall morning.

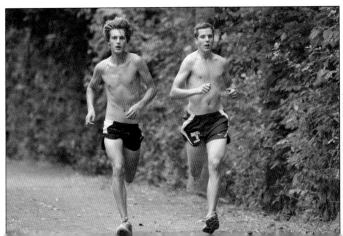

: Alison Wade

176

Stay Cool

To mitigate the effects of heat on individual runs, there are the obvious ways to lessen dehydration's toll: Run early in the morning or after sunset; wear as little clothing as modesty allows; make sure the clothing encourages sweat to evaporate instead of trapping it; moderate your pace from the outset. This is all basic common sense, but in some cases is easier said than done, especially on the timing aspect. Most workdays you're going to have to run when you can, and make the best of it.

Research has shown benefits to precooling before running in hot weather. That research was conducted on subjects wearing ice vests, but it has applicability for the rest of us. If you're able to be in a supercooled environment, like a closed room with the air-conditioning cranked, in the 15 minutes before you run, your core temperature should drop a bit. That should allow you to run farther before dehydration becomes a limiting factor.

177

To Drink or Not to Drink

On most summer runs in most locales, you don't need to carry water. You can do whatever you want, of course, but your sweat losses on an average 45-minute run on an average summer day aren't going to significantly affect your performance. I'm with most longtime runners in preferring to err on the side of a little too much dehydration over having the feel of a run marred by a fuel belt or bottle in hand.

The exceptions would be when working harder or longer than usual. If you're doing a hard workout, even if not on a track, you're probably frequently passing the same spot, such as the bottom of a hill you're doing repeats on. It's easy to stash a bottle there to sip from during your recovery jogs. You'll be sweating more than usual because of a higher work output. Also, because your goal in the workout is to sustain higher-end performance, you'll want to do what you can to keep your sweat losses below the threshold where you're forced to slow significantly.

On long runs, simply being out there twice as long as usual means you're probably going to slow toward the end unless you can recoup some of your sweat losses. Start your weekend long runs early if necessary, and plan a route that has you passing a couple times a spot where you've placed a bottle.

Research has shown that sport drinks at the proper concentration (about 6–8 percent) rehydrate you as fast as water, while providing the additional benefit of sodium, which helps your blood maintain its proper balance.

178
In Between Hot Runs

After any run when you've lost more than 2 percent of bodyweight to sweat, you need to start rehydrating immediately. Delaying doing so will delay your recovery. It used to be thought that you needed to stagger your drinking to properly rehydrate;

most people's internal organs, it was said, couldn't process more than 7–8 ounces of fluid every 15 minutes. It's now been shown that's not true. If you get done running and want to gulp down a quart of water or sport drink, go for it.

Away from the immediate aftermath of a hot run, you still need to be thinking like a runner. Chronic dehydration is the real consistency sapper in the summer. It's easy to slightly underhydrate a few days in a row, after which you'll start to notice feeling lethargic and unmotivated. If at any time during a hot spell your urine is medium to dark yellow, you're not properly rehydrating during the day.

One nice thing to keep in mind is that research has shown that runners who are acclimated to hot-weather training perform better in not only hot weather (duh) but also cooler weather. Heat training, it turns out, has some of the performance-enhancing benefits of altitude training. Two takeaways from this: First, keeping at your running during a long, hot stretch will pay big dividends in the fall. Second, if you're forced to go slower than usual most days, you're still advancing your fitness, just like slower runs at altitude provide more of a training stimulus than might seem the case while you're doing them.

179

Warming to Winter Running

The "You run in this?" query comes more often in winter than summer. But running in sub-freezing temperatures isn't really that big of a deal after the first 10 minutes. By then blood flow to your muscles is significantly increased, and you feel a lot warmer. I always dress for what I'm going to feel like 15 minutes into the run than for the first few steps out the door. I'd rather be a little chilled at first than be weighed down with extra clothing half an hour later, when I'm moving well and probably no longer thinking about the temperature.

The exception for most people is their hands, which seldom warm as much as your core. But they do usually get a bit warmer, and mittens can sometimes make your hands start sweating. I have a pair of gloves with a fold-over mitten flap that's the perfect solution for this problem.

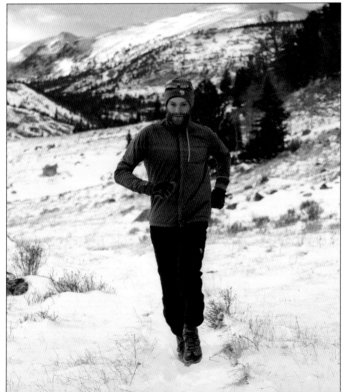

: Joel Wolpert

180

Winter Wear

It's rare to need more than a couple of layers up top. There's so much high-quality cold-weather gear on the market these days that it's hard to go wrong as long as you go with the goods from a well-known company. I've become a big fan of merino wool gear, which insulates fantastically at a wide range of temperatures and doesn't stink even after several runs.

Down below, the biggest concern is keeping the family area warm. I've done a polar bear dip in which I submerged myself in the ocean in Maine on a cold, windy New Year's Day. The discomfort of that was nothing compared to what I've felt the last few miles of and the first half hour after longish runs on brutally cold days. On really cold runs (under 15 degrees) or it's especially windy, I wear wool briefs. Nylon ones with a protective panel in the crotch also work well.

181

Got Traction? Running on Snow

Running on snowy and/or icy roads has gotten a lot easier in recent years with the wide availability of traction devices you can attach to your shoes, such as YakTrax and STABILicers. They allow you to run with much more normal mechanics than would be the case in just your running shoes.

The first time I ran in YakTrax, I was dubious. My run was fine, and I certainly felt like my form wasn't the usual slip-sliding-away phenomenon that can make running on snow so unenjoyable. But I wanted to be sure I wasn't imagining things, so when I got home, I took off the YakTrax and then ran down my street in just my shoes. The difference was obvious. Now I wear them or STABILicers whenever I know the bulk of my run is going to be on roads that haven't been plowed to the pavement. I've also worn them in the woods once I know trails have been heavily traversed by hikers and snowshoers, resulting in a firm surface. It's a real treat to run on favorite trails at a time of year they would otherwise be inaccessible.

If you run on snowy roads without one of these traction devices, expect your hamstrings, especially at their insertion points below your butt, to be sore afterward. Your iliotibial bands are also likely to get aggravated from the extra work they'll do to stabilize you with every step. Do some gentle stretching of those areas after snowy runs, and then apply ice for a few minutes to the top of your hamstrings.

182

Running After Dark

For most people, running throughout the year is going to mean some stretches of running in the dark. Months on end of this isn't the greatest thing ever—which perhaps explains the lack of great marathoners from the Arctic Circle—but running in the dark does have its charms. Seeing where you're going usually isn't an issue, the major exception being bad footing in wintry conditions. Black ice is hard to finesse your way through and probably a good time to look for a treadmill.

The more important matter is usually making sure you're seen by others, by which I mean drivers. Most winter running gear, and many shoes, have reflective materials on them. Get some. If the roads where you run are especially narrow or your local drivers above-and-beyond distracted, go with extra hey-I'm-over-here items, like a reflective vest or a headlamp. You can even buy lights that wrap around your hands like a pair of illuminated brass knuckles (which may be tempting to use when yet another driver jabbering away on his phone acts like you're the one causing the safety hazard).

183

Running in Rain

In most cases the biggest issue with rain is psychological—there's just something about heading out into a downpour that's so much worse than if the rain were to start falling once you're out. I always try to remind myself that you can get only so wet, and you'll reach that state of saturation within the first 10 minutes.

If it's a cold rain, there's no getting around it—the run is unlikely to be one of the highlights of your life. That's one of the few times I dress for how it's going to feel stepping out the door, because even if you do warm up, your clothes will be drenched by then, so a little bit of extra weight won't really matter.

I always make sure my shoes are tied snugly when it's raining. If they're too loose, the rain is going to cause your feet to slip around some, and your knees or other parts of your leg can get achy before the run is over from the extra motion.

184
Withstanding the Wind

The main thing with wind is the annoyance factor. It can be impossible to feel smooth and relaxed if the wind is too strong, even if you're running with a tailwind. The common advice on windy days is to head out into the wind so that you're not facing a headwind on the way home, because that could chill you. I think the opposite approach is better. I sort of trick myself into staying out for longer than I otherwise would on horribly windy days by heading out with the wind at my back. Once it's time to turn around and head home, I'm x number of miles away and have no choice but to finish the job. (And by then I've warmed up.) I'm much more likely to get in a decent amount of mileage that way then willing myself through the opening miles into a headwind, when I'm not yet in a groove.

185
Love, Hate, and Treadmills

Some runners love treadmills, some hate them. I'm more in the latter camp, although I definitely appreciate them at times. I have one in my garage, and just knowing it's there is a source of comfort. Blizzard coming tomorrow? Not my first choice of offerings from the weather gods, but I know I'll still get a run in, either outside if things aren't totally ridiculous, or on the treadmill if I decide that overall my experience will be better by staying inside.

If running on a treadmill is going to mean you run on days that you otherwise wouldn't, then have at it. I've certainly had winter runs where afterward I grudgingly acknowledge I've chosen incorrectly and would have had a more positive experience by hitting the treadmill. There's no denying the safety factor of the treadmill in bad weather winter, especially if you would otherwise be running in the dark with uncertain footing.

186
Treadmill or Dreadmill?

The obvious issue with treadmill running is boredom. This is a rare instance where people who don't really like running probably have an advantage—if it's drudgery to them whether they're outside or on the treadmill, they don't have to employ any special mental armor to stay on the treadmill long enough to make it worthwhile. If, on the other hand, you really love the feel of running over the earth, the breeze in your face, the passing scenery, then treadmill running feels like having to make do with a poor substitute. (I always think of a heavy Scotch drinker being told, "Here, you can have as much light beer as you want, but nothing else.")

Music via something like an iPod is the go-to solution here, especially if you're on a gym treadmill. There is evidence to support running to music with a faster tempo, around 180 beats per minute, so that the feel of the music is in sync with a typical running cadence. At home, TV shows or movies can help the time pass quicker. Really, do whatever it takes to step outside that part of your brain that keeps staring at the console thinking, "Twelve minutes?!? It feels like I've been on here for an hour!"

187
Should You Grade Your Treadmill?

Whether to set the treadmill at a grade is a source of endless debate. Legendary coach and exercise physiologist Jack Daniels has long recommended setting treadmills at a 1 percent grade to account for the fact that you're not overcoming wind resistance, as you would outside. That slight elevation, he claims, results in the same "cost" of oxygen consumption as running the same pace outside on flat ground.

Others doubt the relevance of that issue, and add this question to their objection: Why not just set the treadmill at a faster pace? That is, instead of saying, "I'll put the treadmill at a 1 percent grade and my normal pace," why not keep the grade at 0 percent and set the speed a little faster? That way, not only do your running mechanics feel more normal, but you slightly reduce your time on the treadmill.

I like to mix it up throughout a treadmill run, sometimes with the grade at 0 percent, sometimes at 1 percent, sometimes much steeper. This variety makes a treadmill run more like a "real" run, with its frequent ups and downs and flat stretches.

188
Ignore Your Treadmill Console

Don't place too much stock in the treadmill console's numbers. Hopefully, you can trust the clock and grade setting, but the chances that the treadmill is perfectly calibrated are slim to none in most settings. Certainly don't freak out that you're in horrible shape if the treadmill console is telling you that what you thought was your normal training pace feels really hard. Conversely, don't get overly confident about your fitness for outdoor races if your treadmill is telling you you're doing mile repeats far faster than ever. As much as you can in such an artificial setting, base how fast you go on the treadmill on what feels right for the day, regardless of what pace the console claims that is.

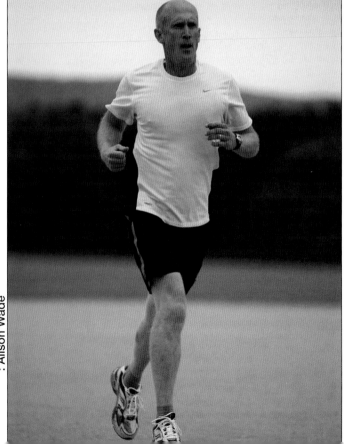

: Alison Wade

189
After the Last PR

It's easy to stay fired up about your running when you feel like your fastest days are still ahead of you. Maintaining consistency gets harder, however, when you realize that you've set your last personal best, that no matter what you do, the most you can hope for in performance terms is to slow the rate of slowing.

The age at which that happens varies greatly. Most new runners can expect to improve for 10–12 years if they're consistent with their running from the start. So a longtime runner who ran on her high school track team might hit her competitive peak in her late twenties, then plateau, then start to slow a bit, then start to slow more dramatically in her late thirties and early forties. If you're an adult-onset runner, you can count on continued improvement for several years at the beginning of your running career, even if you're moving from your forties to your fifties during that time. At some point, however, the effects of aging are going to mean you're on the down slope of the performance curve.

By then, of course, you've probably figured out the things you love most about running and have learned what you need to do to ensure consistency. At the same time, it can be frustrating to think that you're going to get slower and slower for the rest of your running career, and tempting to significantly lessen running's place in your life. Here are a few ways to keep hope alive.

190

Mentally Reboot Frequently

It's easier said than done, but at some point you need to stop comparing yourself to the runner you were at your peak. There's no motivation to come from thinking, "Wait a minute, my pace for a 10K race is now slower per mile than what I used to do on tempo runs."

The best way to avoid thinking like that is to consider the faster, younger you a different runner. At your peak, you probably didn't think, "Wait a minute, my pace for a 10K race is slower per mile than what Runner X does on her easy days." You were motivated by seeing what you could do with the current you and whatever raw material genetics, training history, available time, and other factors gave you to work with. That was true then, and it should be true now. Many successful runners wipe the slate clean every five years. They strive to be the best they've ever been while someone in the 50–54 age group. What they achieved as a forty-eight-year-old

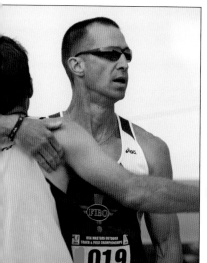

informs their running, for sure, but it doesn't determine their satisfaction with what they're doing now.

One great way to bolster your motivation is to focus on different events or goals. If you were a marathoner in your prime, become a miler for a year. If you concentrated on short races when run-

: 101° West

ning fast felt easy, then see what you can do in long trail races. Find personally meaningful new goals—and they don't have to be race goals—that take you in a different direction.

191

Mentally Reboot Your Calendar As Well

Every ambitious older runner will tell you that recovery between hard or long workouts takes longer than it did at their peak. Whereas at one point you may have needed only one easy day after a track workout before being ready for a good tempo run, now you might need two or three days until you're ready to go hard again.

This change can be easy to accept mentally, but difficult to satisfyingly implement. We all tend to think in terms of seven-day cycles, even though that has no meaning to our bodies. As an

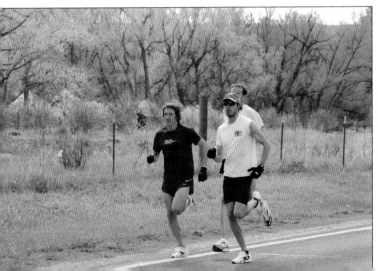

: Brian Metzler

older runner aiming to maintain consistent good training that has momentum, try to move away from tying your training to calendar weeks. For logistical reasons, of course, it's easy to maintain some of your old patterns, such as doing your long runs on Sundays. That's especially the case if you have regular training partners. But at some point you're going to make more progress by not cramming the elements of a good training program into the artificial construct of a seven-day week.

Think in terms of larger blocks of time, like a month. Map your training by deciding what key runs you want to do in that month, and then plan to do them in a logical pattern that accounts for the extra recovery you need as an older runner. That very well might result in a hard workout on Thursday of one week and Tuesday the following. Long-term, you'll build greater momentum this way, and that momentum will help fuel a positive-feedback cycle of motivation.

192

Don't Get Injured

Avoiding injury is crucial for all runners seek consistency, but it's mandatory for older runners. Slower recovery time with age means that an Achilles flare-up that might have been a 48-hour affair in your twenties now drags on for weeks. And if you have to miss some days of running, the return is much harder for a fifty-year-old than someone half her age. You simply can't afford to lose time to injury when one of the main aims of your running is to ward off the effects of time.

193

Build Your Running Body

Maintaining or, better yet, increasing flexibility and muscle strength is crucial for older runners. Those contributors to good running will decline with age unless tended to. Staying strong and supple will not only help you resist injury. As an older runner, you'll simply feel more like your former self. That feeling alone, of running being a flowing, pleasurable activity, will be a massive motivator.

194

Stay Speedy

It's normal as an aging runner to shift away from fast running to something more like a senior shuffle. Avoid that. Regular small doses of fast running will decrease, not increase, your risk of injury. They'll help you maintain muscle mass and range of

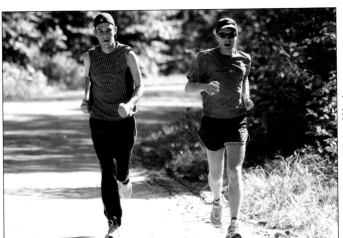

: Alison Wade

motion through the full running stride, and will keep your central nervous system capable of operating at a higher level. Frequency is more important than volume here—6 to 10 20-second bursts at the pace you could hold for 3 minutes, twice a week after an easy run, will do wonders.

Plus, isn't it fun to feel like a kid, sprinting down the street?

195
The Kids Are All Right

If you can find younger training partners, make an effort to run with them regularly. Being around runners who are still chasing PRs is a wonderful antidote to getting bogged down in a woe-is-me-I'm-so-old-and-slow self-pity party. You can feed off of their enthusiasm, and you can put your hard-earned wisdom to use in mentoring them. Several friends of mine have found their running reborn by coaching and running with high schoolers.

196
Travel Regulations

Consistent running is one thing when you're home and in your routine, another when you're traveling for work or pleasure.

Always get a run in before getting on an airplane. Even if it means a token few miles too early in the morning, you'll be glad you did something good for yourself before surrendering your fate to the vagaries of air travel. If it works out that you can get in another run upon arrival, great, but never plan on it.

If you have to get up super early for a flight, then a little less sleep from waking a bit earlier to run won't matter. (Besides, you're going to be on a plane all day! What does it matter if you're a little groggy?) I've had runs I'll remember for the rest of my life—toward the sounds of the Mendenhall Glacier in the dark in Juneau, Alaska, around Nehru Park in New Delhi, India, at 3:30 AM—because of this approach. No way would I trade those runs for a little more sleep before a long travel day.

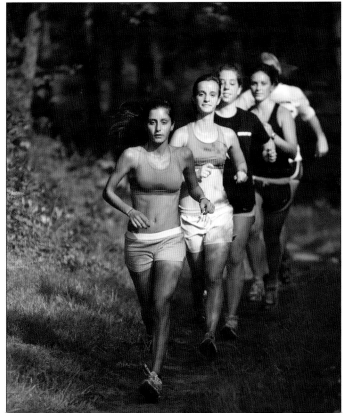

: Alison Wade

197

Packing: Always Be Ready to Run

Running gear goes in your carry-on luggage. The more exotic your location, the greater the chance your checked baggage won't meet you at the airport, and the lesser the chance you'll be able to quickly get replacement items once you're there. I have a friend who put her running gear in her checked luggage for a two-week trip to Africa that occurred while she was deep in preparation for a marathon. Her luggage, including her running shoes, showed up at her hotel with just two days to go in her trip.

At the least, bring your running shoes and one outfit appropriate to your destination's weather onboard with you.

198

Why Wouldn't You Run on Vacation?

I've never understood people who don't run on vacation. Running is something that makes my life better, that refreshes me, that broadens my horizons. Aren't these some of the main reasons people go on vacation?

I tend to run more, not less, when on vacation. Longtime runners know there's no better way to really get a feel for a place than exploring it on the run. You'll see how the locals really live, what the rhythm and aura of the place is really like, the special spots that probably aren't on tourist maps. You'll almost certainly find better places to eat than what your hoteliers will tell you.

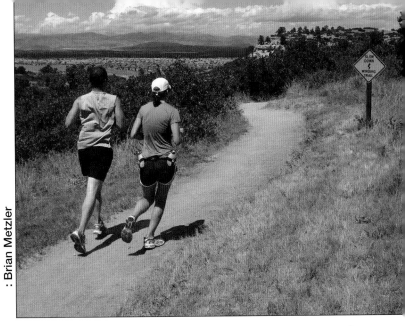

: Brian Metzler

If the people you're on vacation with have the endearing habit of wanting to spend the day with you, simple: Get up a little early and get your run in before the day's sightseeing. In many busy tourist areas, you'll have the streets to yourself early in the morning.

199

Morning Business

If you're traveling for work rather than pleasure, you'll almost always increase your chances of success by running in the morning. Between meetings that run long and working lunches and obligatory cocktail hours, it can be tough to slip out for a run once others have claim on your time.

200

Runner in a Strange Land

Look for bike paths and parks while you're making your way to your hotel and again online once you're situated and have your bearings. At the worst, you can almost always find a short loop or quiet neighborhood to do repeated rounds of. Think of hotel treadmills as a last resort—get out and see the world!

Local running clubs are a great source for finding the best places to run. Even if you can't meet the group for a run, write before you travel and ask the local experts where the hidden gems of a route are.

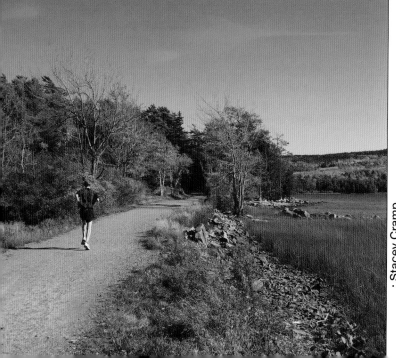

: Stacey Cramp

201

Final Thought on Running Consistently

Behavioral economists talk about the importance of choice architecture, or the environment in which we make choices. The classic example is the difference between an employer-matched retirement fund where participation requires choosing to enroll versus enrollment being the default option. In the latter case, more employees participate. The gist of the field's teaching is: Make it easy to do the right thing.

Choice architecture is huge for daily and long-term success in running. Whether it's anticipating when you'll be able to run tomorrow, or regularly placing yourself in the company of other runners, or spending a little extra for a hotel near a park, make good choices about the overall environment in which your running occurs. Make it easy to do the right thing for your running.

~

PART FIVE

Running Miscellany: 49 Tips on Shoes and Safety, Attitude and Altitude, and Everything Else That Matters

202
It Doesn't Always Get Worse

When you hit a rough spot on a run, remind yourself: It doesn't always get worse. Our bodies are mysterious things, and you can go from feeling fine to poor to great within just a few miles. Finding yourself struggling for the last few minutes doesn't mean that the rest of your run is destined to continue to deteriorate.

If the rough spot continues on for longer than a few minutes, back off the pace and see if that helps. Often, though, the key is to acknowledge the rough spot, do a quick scan to make sure it's nothing serious (like an intestinal issue), and then wait it out. If it's like most rough patches, it too will pass.

Running: The Numbers

Avoid tying your training to arbitrary numbers. As Olympic marathoner Don Kardong once noted in relation to weekly mileage, 88 is a much rounder number than 100. (Besides, can you honestly say that all your courses are precisely calibrated?) This notion also applies to numbers outside of weekly volume. As I noted in chapter 1, "one mile" and "10 percent" are meaningless constructs to your body, so why would "Increase your mileage by no more than 10 percent per week" have any relevance to how you can safely progress? Similarly, 8:00 or 7:00 or whatever number you've decided is the pace per mile at which anything slower is a waste of time might mean something to your head, but not to your body.

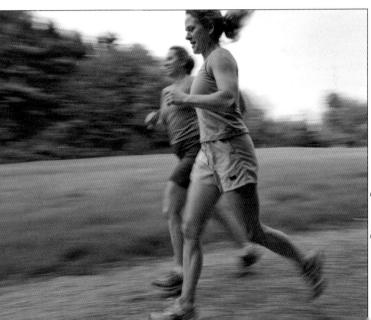

: Stacey Cramp

204

Rise and Shine Before Morning Runs

If you run first thing in the morning, experiment with how much time works best for you between getting up and getting out the door. We all have a perfect amount of time between rising and running that maximizes precious sleep time while allowing the first part of the run to be enjoyable.

With age, most runners find they need more time to feel ready to run. Unless I have to start super early, like at 4:30 before a flight, I get up at least half an hour before I intend to start running. I'd rather get a little less sleep than feel like a zombie the first few miles. That's a great time to do little tasks, like pay bills and see what work e-mails came over the transom overnight, while still having enough time for some pre-run stretching.

205

When You Gotta Go . . .

If you run enough, occasional pit stops are inevitable, and nothing to worry about. If they happen on most runs, however, you should experiment with different foods at different amounts of time before you run. If it seems that you often have to find a bathroom on the run regardless of what and when you eat, it might be time to consult a doctor about irritable bowel syndrome.

206

Transferable Running Virtue:
I'll Make Do

Longtime runners have great experience in plying their trade in less-than-ideal circumstances. Whether it's the weather or a lack of good venues, a head cold or a chafing shirt, things are almost never going to match our mind's eye view of the perfect run. Yet we soldier on and make the best of whatever situation we find ourselves in.

The "I'll make do" mind-set can be transferred from running to most of the rest of your life with great effectiveness. It's one of many good character traits that running encourages and develops. It's one way that, while running may not make us better than other people, it usually makes us better people than we otherwise would be.

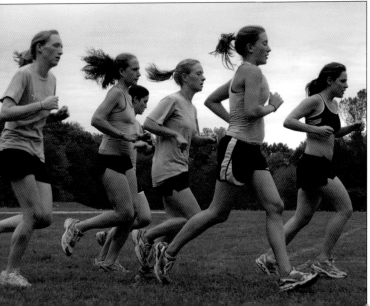

: Alison Wade

207

No Need to "Break In" New Shoes

We used to hear it was necessary to gradually introduce new shoes into your routine, as if shoes were like a new runner who needed to not do too much too soon for fear of breaking down. That's not necessary. Structurally, new shoes should be good right out of the box for however far and fast you want to run in them. (They better be, given their price!)

There's a difference, though, between new shoes and a new model. If your new shoes are fairly different from shoes you've run in recently, then have your first few runs in them be shorter, easier efforts. Two reasons for this: First, to see if they're different enough from what you're used to cause small problems, like irritation across the top of your foot or calf soreness from having a lower midsole. Second, so that if they are initially irksome, you don't ruin a longer, more important run.

But if your new shoes are the same type you've been running in (whether that's the exact same model, an update to an earlier model, or a different brand that's similar in construction to what you're used to), then have at it. I've had 20-milers be a shoe's initiation rite.

208

Shoe Rotation

As your finances allow, it's a good idea to have more than one pair of shoes to run in. Different models will distribute the pounding of running a little differently, so the impact forces will be spread more evenly throughout your body. In theory, rotating shoes should also help individual pairs last longer—midsole materials will have more time to decompress between runs, and the uppers won't disintegrate as readily if they're allowed to fully dry between runs.

If you're going to rotate shoes, stick with the same basic type, such as a lightweight trainer from each of three manufacturers. If you're tied to one brand, they should have models that are related but different enough to result in a slightly different running experience. If you absolutely love one shoe from one manufacturer and it's undeniably the shoe for you, have two or more pairs at various stages of wear. Even those slight differences will lead to different distribution of some impact forces.

209
Shoe Drying 101

The best way to dry your shoes after a rainy run? Remove the insoles and then stuff the shoes with crumpled-up newspaper. Wrap more newspaper around the insoles. If it's been an

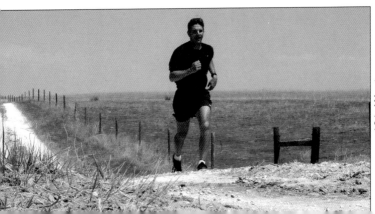

: 101° West

especially drenching run, you might have to restuff the shoes once or twice before they're dry. Unfortunately, I can tell you from personal experience that getting shoes even close to a significant heat source isn't the way to go—the glues and rubber and whatnot rapidly disintegrate and you're left with an unsalvageable shoe.

210
Of Shoe Reviews and Salt

At the risk of committing professional suicide, allow me to suggest that you not rely solely on shoe reviews in running magazines to decide what to buy.

The biggest reason to take magazine shoe reviews with a grain of salt isn't because the magazines are in bed with the manufacturers, who are among their biggest advertisers. If a shoe has design issues, the better running magazines will note that. The reason to not take shoe reviews as gospel stems from the logistics of magazine production: There's simply not enough time between when new shoes become available and when you read about them for magazine wear-testers to put significant miles on them. That short window gets even shorter when you realize the wear-testers probably have several models to try at once. So while they may be able to make valuable comments about the shoe's construction and whether it feels like it's supposed to, they can't speak to the key matter of durability. A shoe could be the greatest shoe in the world but not worth buying if it starts falling apart after 150 miles.

Supplement what you read in shoe reviews with real-world long-term data from fellow runners on a good online forum.

211

Tread Lightly Around In-Store Analysis of Your Running Form

It's become common at specialty running stores to video customers running on a treadmill as a means of helping them choose the right shoe. Don't place too much stock in these analyses.

For starters, most people run slightly differently on treadmills. Second, what they're mostly looking for in these analyses is your degree of pronation, or how much your foot rolls in between initial contact with the ground and toeing off. Concentrating on that one aspect of the running gait as the key to determining optimal shoe choice is an outdated approach. Finally, and I don't mean to be harsh here, but come on: The person doing the analysis could be a twenty-year-old making $10 an hour. He might have the best intentions in the world, but should hardly be taken as your shoe guru.

If you're going to do the treadmill gait analysis, use it as one small bit of information contributing toward your shoe decision. If the salesperson insists on shoehorning you into a model that's significantly different than what you've had success with on the basis of the treadmill analysis, run away.

212

They're Your Shoes, So Have at Them

Running shoes aren't Apple products—you're allowed to alter them to fit your needs. Experiment with different lacing

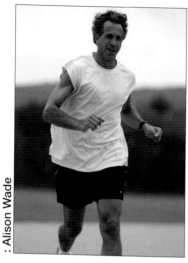

: Alison Wade

techniques to find the one that best results in a snug but comfortable fit. For some people, that's going to mean extra looping at the top eyelets to better hold the heel in place. For others it might mean skipping some of the middle eyelets to better accommodate a high instep or wide forefoot.

Sometimes you'll be inspired to personalize other parts of the shoe, like cutting off the top of the heel counter to lessen irritation on your Achilles tendon. Five years ago, when it seemed all shoes were being made with rigid plastic bridges under the arch, I spent a lot of time hacking away with an X-ACTO knife to remove the plastic and get a more flexible shoe. (Fortunately, for the sake of both my feet and my oft-cut hands, that trend in shoe making has abated.)

213
Transferable Running Virtue: Now Is the Time

Busy modern runners have to fit in their running around a million other claims on their time. Tomorrow morning at 7:00

probably isn't the ideal time for a long tempo run, but that's when it needs to happen, or it is going to happen at all. And guess what? Once you're doing it, and especially once it's over, you'll realize that time was as good as any.

This is running's version of carpe diem. Running can help you approach the rest of your life with that same attitude—now is the time to go do something good. Waiting isn't going to help, because the next hour will have its own challenges.

214
Lessons from (Your) History

Look through your old logs once in a while. Even when you were running PR after PR, things were never as effortless as you now remember them. And when you were hurt or struggling, you got through it, just like you will the next time you hit a roadblock.

215
Running as Commuting

If you can swing it logistically, try running to or from work a couple times a week. Running to work means you get to the office with both run and commute out of the way while being able to sleep later than if you ran first, then commuted. Why, you might even find you're in a good mood for the start of the workday! Running home from work gives you a wonderful way to shed the stress of the workday and walk into your home able to devote your full attention to whatever awaits you there.

The biggest challenge (assuming the distance from home to work is doable) is planning, but that's not much of a barrier. When I had jobs I ran to, I brought in an extra pair of clothes the day before. Depending on how you get to work, running home can mean figuring out a way to get to work the next morning if, say, your car spends the night at the office. (May I suggest running there?) Running home from rather than to work saves you the issue of what to do if there's not a shower at your office.

Running as a means of commuting saves time, money, and frustration. I enjoyed many a morning run on the trails of Washington's Rock Creek Park en route to work as I looked down at a line of cars I was moving faster than.

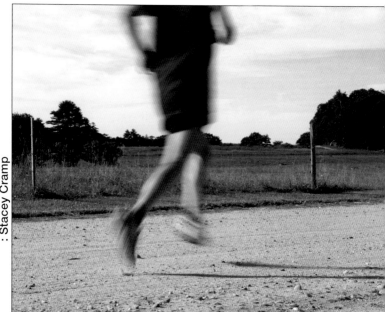

216

Running Errands

Another great way to put your running to functional use is to combine it with errands. The obvious one here is dropping your car off at a garage and running home, and then running to pick it up when it's ready the next day. (Or if your mechanic is like mine, the next week.) But I've known busy runners who have run to the dentist's office or other appointments where their appearance wasn't a primary concern.

217

Know Your Serum Ferritin Level

If you've been feeling unaccountably worn down for at least a few weeks, you could be suffering from iron deficiency. When your iron is low, you'll lose enthusiasm for running and most of your runs will feel like chores. Faster running will be especially difficult; your times for hard workouts and races will get much worse.

It's common when feeling like that to have your blood checked. Trouble is, the measures usually looked at, such as hemoglobin level, can be within the acceptable range, and then you'll start thinking you're a head case or have something much worse wrong with you. Ask to have your serum ferritin level checked; it's usually not included on a standard blood test. Serum ferritin is a measure of your body's iron stores, sort of like the nest egg you're not supposed to touch unless things get dire. It can show problems with iron storage and absorption even if more standard measures of anemia are fine.

If your serum ferritin level is below 30, it's probably affecting your performance. Increase the amount of iron-rich foods in your diet and you should feel better within a month. It's a good idea to have your serum ferritin level measured when you're feeling great in your running. That will give you a baseline to compare to for future readings.

218
Other Medical Matters

Running will cause some benign changes in standard medical tests. Amazingly, some doctors are still unaware of these changes.

The most obvious change is that your resting heart rate gets lower. By now most medical types are aware of this adaptation to endurance exercise, but it's still worth mentioning preemptively. (Although it is fun to sit there with a pulse of 38 and watch the nurse look at her watch as if it's not working.) Long-term running will also cause an increase in your blood volume. Red blood cell production often doesn't keep up with the larger overall blood volume, resulting in hemoglobin and red blood cell counts that could be interpreted as signs of anemia in sedentary people.

Long-term running will also cause two changes to the structure of your heart: the left ventricle wall will get thicker and the entire left ventricle will get larger. In sedentary people, a thickened left ventricle wall can be a precursor to heart attacks and strokes;

a larger left ventricle can signal a leaky heart valve. Be sure your doctor knows you run before any tests are done on your heart.

219

Don't Run to Your Medical Appointment

In the short-term, running, especially hard running, can cause temporary changes in medical measurements that could be taken as signs of disease. For example, after a hard run, your blood

levels of the muscle enzyme creatine phosphokinase will be elevated for a few hours. Increased levels of this enzyme can accompany a heart attack. Similarly, after hard running, your levels of the enzyme aspartate aminotransferase will be elevated; a doctor seeing this is likely to conclude something is wrong with your liver. Avoid these situations by not running hard the day before or of a medical appointment.

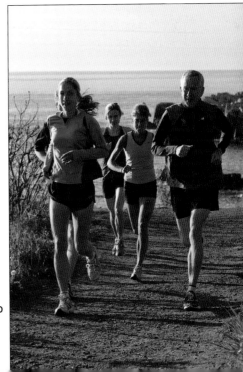

: Stacey Cramp

220

Black-and-White Appeal as You're Graying

One thing to cherish about running, especially as you age, is how you can measure it in clear-cut terms if you want. Did I run faster at last weekend's 5K than on the same course last year? Am I now averaging more miles per week than I was two years ago?

Those objective measures of success are increasingly hard to come by in most other areas of modern life. Are you a better parent than you were five years ago? Are you a better person to be in a relationship with than you used to be? A better friend? How do you know? Even at work, most of us lack quantifiable, black-and-white barometers of progress. We move data around, we have meetings about meetings, we write memos, we serve others, we collaborate. Rewarding work, for sure, but difficult to point at and say, "Yes, here I can see exactly how much I did, and how good it was; others' evaluation of my work doesn't really matter." Running, especially through racing, can offer needed time in the no-spin zone.

221

Wanted: Good Running Partners

Finding people to run with can be a patchwork project, but always worth the effort. Most local running clubs have group runs where you can find people of roughly your current level of fitness. From there you can get to know which ones you mesh with and whose life details could facilitate frequent runs together. (Do they live reasonably near you? Work roughly the same schedule? And so on.)

A great way to meet new running partners is talking with people who finish near you at races. After you give each other the obligatory "nice job" handshake, ask if they want to join you on your cool-down. Could be that the person lives five miles from you and is dying to find others to run with.

222
Transferable Running Virtue: Chip Away

I hope by now I've convinced you that long-term success in running comes via persistence, not paroxysms of effort. That big-picture investor's mind-set works well in most of life as well. As a runner and a person, be the person who chips away at goals methodically, steadily, intelligently.

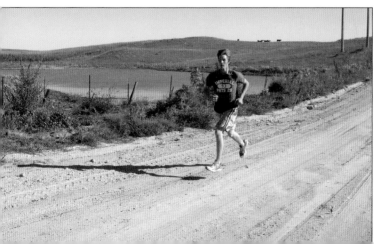

:101° West

223

Embrace Non-Running Exertion

Don't shy away from unplanned, unstructured activity in the rest of your life just because you're a runner. Resting up when not running may have made sense when we all worked in steel mills or on farms, but today the opposite issue is more often the problem—we're sort of in a constant half-slumber from barely moving. I've detailed throughout the book how our sedentary lifestyles compromise our running ability. Here's one more nudge along those lines: Moderate activity soon before running, like gardening, playing with your children, walking the dog, or raking the yard, will serve as a warm-up. It will help to bridge the gap between sitting for hours and running with good form.

If these sorts of moderate activities interfere with a run you do soon after, then you're that much more in need of a good whole-body stretching and strengthening program.

224

Eat and Run

Experiment to find the best balance for you between leaving enough time after eating so that your stomach doesn't bother you when you're running and eating close enough to your run so that you don't feel weak and light-headed. I have the world's wimpiest intestinal system and usually run into trouble if I eat within five hours of a run. Contrast that with a guy I used to run a lot with who would be finishing off a plate of bacon as I arrived at his house for a 2-hour run. You'll probably be somewhere between those extremes.

If you start runs feeling a little light-headed and still feel that way 15 minutes into it, then you'll probably benefit from having some calories closer to your run. A couple hundred calories of an easily digested food, like bananas or a plain bagel, will help boost your blood-sugar level so that you feel stronger in the first part of your run.

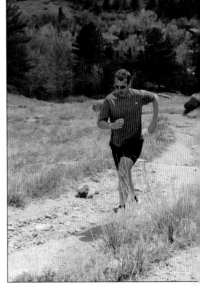

: Brian Metzler

225
How's Your Balance?

Having good balance will make your running more enjoyable. Consider that every running step essentially involves balancing on one foot while moving. When your balance is poor, you introduce a little instability with each step; that can make you slower or fatigued earlier than necessary or even lead to compensation elsewhere that can cause injury. Poor balance becomes a more acute problem when you're running on snow or even on trails, where an inability to right yourself can lead to an injurious fall. Also, poor balance in runners often stems from weak glute muscles, so is a sign that you're not running with as powerful a stride as you could be.

You should be able to stand on one foot and draw the other foot close to your waist and tie your running shoes. If you can't, work to improve your balance. That can be done as simply as by standing on one leg when you brush your teeth in the morning, then on the other leg when you brush your teeth at night. A running-specific strengthening routine like I wrote about in part 3 will also help, as will work on devices like a wobble board.

226
Trail Running Technique

When you run trails, there's a balance to strike between gawking at your beautiful surroundings and staring at the ground to avoid tripping. Regular trail running improves your proprioception, or your sense of your body's placement in space. With more trail running, you get a better instinctual feel for obstacles on the ground and how to run on, over, or around them. Improved proprioception, like improved balance, should help all of your running, especially when

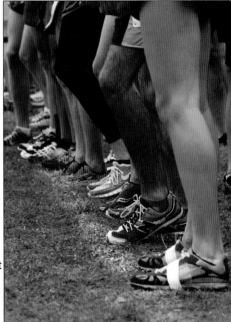

: Joel Wolpert

you're running in the dark and lack as many visual cues about your surroundings.

On trails, run with a light, quick stride that's a bit shorter than you would use on flat, unencumbered terrain.

A good running shoe is a good running shoe, period, and should work fine on most trails. Some people like to wear sturdier shoes on trails, but I think the opposite approach makes more sense—you want a light, low-to-the-ground shoe that will increase your agility. It's the same rationale as choosing minimalist orienteering shoes over high, heavy hiking boots for walks in the woods.

227
Trail Running Times

Leave all your type-A runner mind-set at the trailhead. Disregard concerns that you're going too slow to get in a good workout or that you don't know how far you're going. If ever there's a time to simply lose yourself in the pleasure of running through nature, it's when you're on a nice trail.

228
When the Love of Your Life Doesn't Love Your Running

This can be a tough one. For whatever reason (guilt? jealousy? resentment?), some runners' partners don't like our sport. If that's your situation, do your best to articulate calmly why running is important to you. Describe how it improves your physical and mental well-being, and how your health is important to your future together. If time away from home is an issue, offer to do at least some of your runs when they won't interfere as much with home life. Also offer to regularly spend time together on something that's important to your partner.

Here's a story that I'm hopeful some non-running partners can relate to: One summer in college I found myself at an older runner's house late afternoon for a run together. While he changed out of his work clothes, I talked with his wife. My friend was coming back from an injury and had recently come home from work every day and sat around the house instead of going running. His wife told me how, before he was injured, she resented his running and the time it took away from their relationship. When he got injured, however, she couldn't wait for him to get out of the house and leave her alone! Once he was injured, she realized that his running time had also become her alone time for the day, and she missed it as much as he did his running.

229
Streaking Runners in Perspective

If consistency in running is the key to long-term success, does that mean that having a running streak of never missing a day is the logical conclusion? For almost everyone, no. There are some injuries and non-running conditions and situations where squeezing in a token run shows you've lost sight of the big picture.

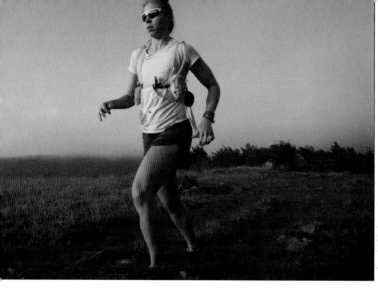

I have a good friend who has run at least 2 miles every day since August 1982, and even he would tell you there have been times an injury would have healed much faster if he had broken his streak.

That said, there's much to be learned from streakers. They always find a way to get it done, showing that the "I don't have time" excuse is usually bunk. And for most of them, their seeming fanaticism has a built-in moderation: You don't run every day for twenty years unless you're really good at reading your body and taking a long-term view. My friend the streaker has run a 2:15 marathon, so it's hard to say that running every day kept from reaching his potential.

I've had a few sizable streaks, the longest one being a bit more than six years. My favorite one wasn't the longest. It was a recent one of more than two years that I ended when a calf problem wasn't improving. I liked that streak because it just sort of happened organically—in those two years there wasn't a day when I was injured or sick enough not to feel like running.

230

Be a Running Ambassador

Be conscious of the fact that others will partly base their opinions of runners on you. We're not the only ones on the roads and trails. Always try diplomacy first with irritants like people walking in the inside land of the track or unleashed dogs.

231

Counsel on Coaches

If you decide you want to work with a coach, do your homework on the person. Ask to communicate with other runners she's coached. Find out how long people are usually coached by him and why they no longer are. Most important, find out how individualized an approach she takes. Will the training you're given be tailored to your running background, your goals, your rest-of-life situation? How often will you be allowed to call or write when you have questions or hit a rough few days?

If you get the sense that you're being given the same program everyone receives, you could do just as well with a good running book or an online library of workouts.

232

If You Find Yourself at Altitude

Run! You're in for an interesting experience.
If you're suddenly plopped down (well, up) at 5,000 feet or

more of elevation, start your runs exceedingly gently. If you start a run too fast at sea level, you can recover once you realize your mistake and salvage an enjoyable run. At altitude, you'll probably remain hurting the rest of the run. And given that the hurting takes the form of feeling like you're being strangled and that your legs are about to collapse Gumby-like under you, it's best to avoid it.

Once you're warmed up, you'll probably feel better your first day or two at altitude than on, say, the fifth day. On the early days, you're not yet worn down from the new stress of being at altitude. Later in the week, you won't yet have

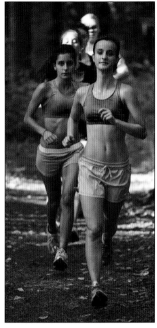

: Alison Wade

acclimated (that will take at least a week) but will be dealing with cumulative fatigue.

Expect to feel particularly challenged on uphills. If you don't let your breathing get completely out of control, you should be able to recover relatively quickly once you get to flat ground or a blessed downhill stretch.

Drink more water than usual, or your cumulative fatigue after a few days will be compounded. Headaches are a sign that you're not adequately rehydrating.

If you're going to be at altitude for just a few days, don't bother with trying to do your normal hard workouts. Just running slowly will be challenging enough. It's a good idea, however, to do striders every few days if you're not used to running at altitude. A set of 20-second short bursts of fast running will put a little pop in your legs, which will likely otherwise feel sluggish from slogging away in thin air. Take complete recovery between striders at altitude so that you can run each one with light, efficient form and your breathing doesn't become a limiting factor.

233
Let the Children Play

Young runners should run as much as they want to. There's no evidence to support the contention that running as a growing teen will stunt growth. If a teen enjoys her running, is doing it because she wants to, and is continuing to improve while remaining injury-free, she's on the right track. I ran a marathon while in high school and didn't burn out on the sport, as is so often feared for young runners. Thirty years after that marathon, I'm more in love with running than ever.

234
Run Away from Ruts

When you feel like you're in a rut, make a deliberate effort to shake things up. It doesn't take much to make a run feel fundamentally different. Something as simple as doing one of your normal loops in the opposite direction will have you seeing

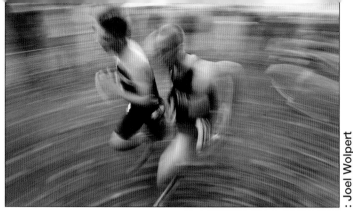

familiar sights anew. Even better, head out the door without the slightest plan of where to run, and see where your instincts lead you. Run down a street you've always avoided, just so you can say to yourself, "Hey, today I ran somewhere I've never run before."

Sometimes you need to take more drastic (but still simple) steps to jump-start things. Run at an unusual time of day. Run with someone a lot slower than yourself to experience what running is like for them. Run with someone a lot faster to see how long you can hang on.

One of the best ways to get out of a running funk is to drive to run somewhere different. Even driving a couple miles from home, so that you're running on familiar ground but from a novel starting place, makes a run feel different. You can also run somewhere, like to a coffee shop where someone will meet you with fresh clothes and an espresso. Or if you're out running errands with someone, give them your civilian clothing and run home.

Here's my last-resort technique for when I need a run to feel different: Wear crazy clothes. I've gone topless in ridiculously baggy basketball shorts and find it impossible not to occasionally look down at what I'm running in and laugh. You usually need just one out-of-the-ordinary run to mentally reboot and realize how much you like running.

235

The World Can Wait

Except in extenuating circumstances like being on call for work or an ongoing family crisis, leave your phone at home when you run. Let your running time be a sanctioned break from always being plugged in. Use the time to clear your head to be that much more effective when you do return to the world of constant contact.

236

Yond Cassius Has a Lean and Hungry Look

If you were healthy and at a good weight when you were twenty five, there's almost never a good reason to be significantly heavier than that.

People like to tell themselves they've added muscle over the years, about which two things: First, come on, that's usually not the case. Second, to the extent that people do add muscle as they age, it's often to support their bones, ligaments, and tendons to help deal with the more likely source of increased weight, fat. So even in that case, the extra muscle isn't going to help you run faster.

As runners, we already live in ways contrary to accepted beliefs on what aging is supposed to be like. Why not take that attitude toward weight as well?

237

Sedentary Now ≠ Running Future

How you feel while getting dressed to run is no guarantee of how you'll feel 15 minutes into it. Don't preemptively defeat yourself mentally by projecting from a sedentary state how you'll feel once you get some blood pumping and a pleasant breeze on your face.

238

Midday Dashes

If you run during your lunch hour, you'll probably (and understandably) want to maximize your running time. It's natural in that scenario to skimp a bit on good post-run habits. Do your best once back at work to move around frequently. At your desk, do little stretches throughout the afternoon, such as foot circles or sitting with one foot on the opposite knee and leaning forward for a glute stretch. After dinner, try to get in a more solid stretching session of 10 to 15 minutes so that you're in a better place for the next day's noontime run.

239

Transferable Running Virtue: Endure

If there's one thing we runners do, it's endure. We endure through long runs and hard workouts, weeks of bad weather, and days of

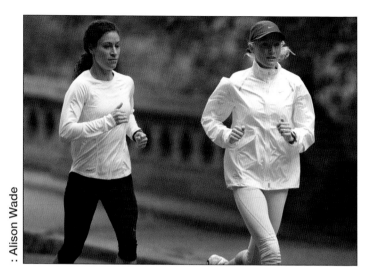

: Alison Wade

low energy. We do what it takes to see things through to the end. We can achieve amazing things in the rest of our lives by practicing that virtue in our non-running endeavors.

240

Stay Flexible (Not Just Muscularly)

Always be open to new running experiences. Who knows what aspects of the sport will appeal to you at different times in your running career? After all, have you always liked the same kind of music, watched the same kind of movies, eaten the same foods, read the same kind of books? Keeping an open mind about the many possible ways to be a runner will increase the chances of finding ones that speak to you for where you are now. Maybe you'll learn that you love running with a group, or that you were born to run on trails, or that you're really a sprinter.

241

Safe Crossings

When you're unsure if a driver at a stop sign sees you and are wondering if it's safe to go about your business, look at the wheels of the tires. You'll notice motion there before anywhere else.

242

Let the Idiot Drivers Yell

I say this as someone who has banged on a car and then been chased by the occupants: It's not worth it. Even if, as is usually the case, the driver is the one at fault in a driver-runner contretemps, let it go. You're not going to change the driver's mind about the situation, you're allowing the driver's irrationality to have too much of an effect on your run and you really don't want to find out that you've pushed some nutcase over the edge while he's operating a two-ton vehicle. If you must have some satisfaction from the encounter, kill him with kindness—when he honks and shakes his fist, smile and wave.

Similarly, it's not worth it to respond to the too many people (usually male teens) who are entertained by shouting supposed insults at passing runners. Even more so than with a potentially distracted driver, you're dealing here with people acting irrationally. (If they were being rational, why would their supreme intended insult be to yell, "Faggot!" As if sexual orientation has any connection to the fact that you're running down the street.) Returning their taunt is just giving them the attention they want.

243
It's Nice to Have Level Hips

When it's safe to do so, switch sides of the road throughout runs so that the same leg isn't always a little lower. Running like that too much can tilt your pelvis and set off a cascade of undesirable compensations. Running both and against traffic is safest on roads with wide shoulders on runs in daylight.

On a particularly sloped road, I'll run toward the middle if I know it's a road that doesn't get much traffic. On those quiet roads, your acquired runner's hearing will alert you in time that you need to get over to one side.

244
Nobody Likes a One-Stepper

When you're running with others, don't be the annoying person who's always ever so slightly ahead of everyone else, a.k.a. a one-stepper. Doing so has an insidious way of putting people on edge, and it often contributes to the pace escalating incrementally on what should be a nice, relaxed social run.

As a reformed one-stepper, I know that you can be one without knowing it until you're told by irritated running partners. Now I'm always conscious that my shoulders aren't two, then three, then four inches ahead of my running partner's.

It's especially uncourteous to one-step when you're running with someone a lot slower than you. Make that person's run a more positive experience by letting him get out in front and set the pace. If you find your momentum carrying you more toward your normal pace, ease back on the throttle and save it for your next solo run.

245

Nobody Likes a Martyr

The quickest way to get others to not take interest in your running is to always be bitching about it. Yes, sometimes it's tiring, or the weather's bad, or you're slower than you were a few years ago, or it seems to take up too much of your time, or you just don't feel like doing it. Sorry, but almost nobody cares. The few who do will, in moments of kindness, indulge your complaints if those complaints are occasional; that's what friends are for. But if your main presentation of your running to others is a litany of

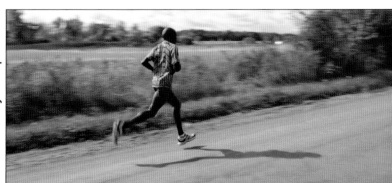

: Stacey Cramp

one insult from the universe after another, they're going to stop listening, and with good reason. (And if they're not runners, why would they ever want to be, given the way you describe it?)

Running is a gift we give ourselves because we realize it makes our lives better. Try to be a good presenter of that gift.

If your image to yourself of running is indeed primarily negative, then you need to explore other elements of the sport and find more of them that appeal to you.

246
Four Key Words for Running

As far as I can tell, A. Lou Vickery, author of books on baseball and more, isn't a runner. But he sure sounds like he knows what it takes to make it in our sport. Here's a choice quote from him: "Four short words sum up what has lifted most successful individuals above the crowd: a little bit more. They did all that was expected of them and a little bit more."

At some point, almost all runners who have reached their potential have been the ones who did what seems like plenty, and a little bit more—a couple extra miles, two more hill repeats, an extra stretching session instead of spending that time playing video games.

247
Running Through Data Smog

Thirty years ago in running, information scarcity was more the issue than information overload. The latter is now a potential stumbling block—everyone with access to blogging software can pronounce himself an expert. As a result, curious runners can be excused if they often feel like they're doing laps around the Tower of Babel.

When trying to wade your way through the glut of running info available online, bear in mind that running is essentially a conservative sport. By that I mean that thousands of runners have tested every theory using the ultimate lab of trial and error out on the roads. If something were "revolutionary" or "the secret," then you can bet that ambitious runners will have investigated it and decided whether it's worth paying attention to from this simple standpoint: Two months later, is my running better because of this? So if some training "secret" that's in contrast to what most good runners do is being presented by someone with no real credentials, pay no attention to that man behind the curtain.

248
At the Risk of Making You Discount This Book

Don't believe everything you read. It is indeed possible to run—long and fast, for months on end—on a stress fracture. (Not that you should, of course.) Rest doesn't cure all injuries. Great races are possible when you're deep into heavy training. Less is almost never more. And here's the real upender: Marathon world record-holder Haile Gebrselassie jogs in place at stoplights.

249

An Important Note About Your Morning Coffee

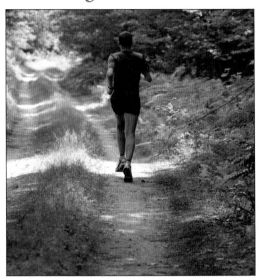

Don't leave the house until the coffee has left you.

: Alison Wade

250

The Most Important Tip

Relax, it's just running. Of course it can be the most intoxicating, captivating, meaningful part of your life. But it's still just running. Nobody's making you do it, and you're not going to save the world doing it. So find what you enjoy about running, and then follow your bliss.